Habilitation, Health, and Agency

Habilitation, Health, and Agency

A Framework for Basic Justice

Lawrence C. Becker

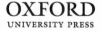
OXFORD
UNIVERSITY PRESS

OXFORD
UNIVERSITY PRESS

Oxford University Press, Inc., publishes works that further
Oxford University's objective of excellence
in research, scholarship, and education.

Oxford   New York
Auckland   Cape Town   Dar es Salaam   Hong Kong   Karachi
Kuala Lumpur   Madrid   Melbourne   Mexico City   Nairobi
New Delhi   Shanghai   Taipei   Toronto

With offices in
Argentina   Austria   Brazil   Chile   Czech Republic   France   Greece
Guatemala   Hungary   Italy   Japan   Poland   Portugal   Singapore
South Korea   Switzerland   Thailand   Turkey   Ukraine   Vietnam

Published by Oxford University Press, Inc.
198 Madison Avenue, New York, New York 10016

www.oup.com

Oxford is a registered trademark of Oxford University Press

Library of Congress Cataloging-in-Publication Data
Becker, Lawrence C.
Habilitation, health, and agency : a framework for basic justice / Lawrence C. Becker.
p.   cm.
Includes bibliographical references (p.   ).
ISBN 978-0-19-991754-9 (acid-free paper) 1. Political science—Philosophy.
2. Justice. 3. Health. 4. Medical ethics. I. Title.
JA79.B35   2012
320.01′1—dc23   2011044543

9 8 7 6 5 4 3 2 1
Printed in the United States of America
on acid-free paper

For Charlotte

Contents

Habilitation, Health, and Agency

Introduction

This book offers a way of reorienting normative theories of distributive justice around conceptions of habilitation, health, and agency. It asks readers for a pause in perennial debates about competing principles of justice in order to consider a constellation of ideas that can reframe the whole theory-building enterprise. If the book achieves its overall aim, it will have described a useful and attractive new conceptual framework for theories of distributive justice generally. It will not have argued for or against any particular normative theory of justice.

The novelty of this conceptual framework—the habilitation framework, as I will call it—lies more in the arrangement and articulation of its parts than in the parts themselves. Those parts (habilitation, basic justice, basic good health, and robustly healthy agency) are reassuringly familiar, taken one by one.

As used here, habilitation is about equipping someone or something with capacities or functional abilities. Basic justice (as opposed to ideal justice) is the most fundamental part of the subject. Basic good health (as opposed to perfect health) is about health fundamentals, but includes psychological as well as physical health. Robustly healthy agency is a strong form of functional competence.

All of this will sound vaguely familiar, but unless it is explicated with some care, the arguments of the book will not be as precise and consistent as they need to be. Such explication begins later in this introduction in "The Plan of the Book and a Short Lexicon for It," and continues as needed. The philosophical argument that flows from these ordinary concepts is much less familiar than the concepts themselves, but the aim here is to make that argument commonsensical: novel, perhaps, but illuminating rather than contentious.

Such common sense is often welcome in ethics. At least that is so in the large area in which all plausible normative theories converge on similar conclusions about right and wrong, good and bad, justice and injustice—even when they disagree about method and first principles. It would be alarming if the habilitation framework offered novel ideas about murder, promise keeping, contracts, cooperation, self-interest, benevolence, and so on—ideas different from settled transcultural and transhistorical social norms, as well as those that libertarians and communitarians, individualists and collectivists, liberals and conservatives, utilitarians and social contract theorists all endorse. Novelty should be more welcome, however, if it is confined to the philosophical considerations that ought to ground such agreement between theories—theories that are otherwise very different in their conceptions of ideal justice, and in utopian visions of it.

So in order to bring out the way in which the habilitation framework applies to normative theories of justice generally, this book will be confined to the area in which they diverge least: basic justice, as I will call it. And readers should not expect to find any new distributive principles proposed here. Rather, the book is about background ideas: material from which distributive principles can be developed, criticized, adopted, applied, revised, refined, or rejected no matter what specific theory of justice one is pursuing.

Three Proposals

The argument of the book yields three overarching proposals for philosophical theories of basic justice: (1) that those theories ought to adopt a particular conception of habilitation as a framing device for their inquiries; (2) that they ought to adopt a particular conception of basic good health as the representative good for basic justice; and (3) that they ought to adopt a specific aspect of health—namely, robustly healthy agency—as the target for basic justice. As a whole, the book is essentially an explication of those concepts and conceptions, together with an argument for the three proposals about them.

Those numbered proposals (and the disclaimer about the deliberate absence of distributive principles) will be repeated throughout the book as canonical statements of its aims, even though many of the terms in them or in the air around them will be initially obscure until the explication of them is complete. "Habilitation," for example, is a particularly challenging case. It is an abbreviation for a complex conception that will have to be developed at considerable length. (It will be given an initial gloss in the short lexicon below, and developed more fully in Chapters 1–2, and 7–8.)

The Absence of Distributive Principles

Notice that these proposals are all about the metric or currency or representative good involved in theories of justice. They are not about any specific list of basic goods, specific ranking of them, or specific distributive principle. In short, they do not give any principled account of how goods ought to be distributed. Nor do they tacitly assume any such principles, or deliberately leave them lurking in the background.

Thus, by extrapolation from Elizabeth Anderson's pithy account of the theoretical necessity for both a metric and a distributive rule in a normative theory of justice (Anderson, 2010, 81–83), the proposals offered here do not constitute such a theory.

As the argument of the book develops, however, it will be natural to wonder whether the proposals in it inadvertently prejudice some choices about normative principles. Such questions will be addressed at various points throughout the text. It is clearly true that the habilitation framework, and the health metric and target projected from it, are likely to make it difficult to justify one or another distributive principle *in a given environment*. But it will turn out that such special difficulties either are attributable to the principles themselves (because they are intrinsically more difficult than others to justify) or are attributable to special features of a given environment.

For example, on the latter point, consider how life on a desolate frontier sparsely populated by nomadic tribes, or in a barely survivable environment (a high-tech colony in Antarctica, or on the moon) might plausibly call for different distributive principles from those best suited for a large-scale, densely populated, affluent, industrialized society. The habilitation framework is sensitive to such environmental variables and thus cannot be expected to impose exactly the same justificatory burdens or benefits on all distributive principles in all environments. What is possible, or even necessary, on a camping trip with a few friends will not always work well when scaled up to a large industrialized society (Cohen, 2009), and if the habilitation framework shifts normative burdens on distributive principles accordingly, that is a good thing.

Antecedents and Analogs

As far as I am aware, no one else has proposed to give habilitation, health, and agency such a central role in theories of distributive justice. Sometimes, one or another of these concepts has played a leading role in a particular normative theory, but that is quite different from giving the three of them leading roles in all theories of justice. And the deliberate omission of distributive principles from this account may make the whole project seem even more peculiar. Is it believable, at this late date, that everyone has so far missed something of central relevance to all theories of justice? Is it worthwhile trying to find something like this rather than getting on with a specific normative enterprise? Such worries may raise eyebrows, if not hackles.

It may help at this point, then, to notice the way in which this book will be analogous to (or even an expanded version of) three familiar preparatory projects that are typically embedded in specific normative theories of distributive justice.

The circumstances of justice. One of these projects is an account of the circumstances of justice—that is, an account of those aspects of the human condition that give rise to questions of justice in the first place, and for the need to theorize about it in some way that can have practical consequences. (Think of Hume's list: moderate scarcity, limited altruism, and approximate equality of power and vulnerability.) There will be an explicit analog to this in Chapter 2, which will describe the circumstances of habilitation for basic justice.

Basic goods. Another familiar project is getting an account of the goods that are especially salient for any theory of distributive justice. (Think of Rawls's preparatory account of basic goods, or Walzer's account of social goods.) There is an analog to such a project here, in the discussion of eudaimonistic health, the health metric, and the healthy agency target—all in Part Two of the book (Chapters 3–6). But identifying goods that are especially salient is not equivalent to giving such goods normative priority. A normative theory may go on to do that, but the habilitation framework will not. It will simply discuss the way in which health and healthy agency are, from a practical point of view, especially useful as a metric and a target, respectively.

The goals of justice. A third analogous project is an account, in very general terms, of the goals of justice—the ultimate goals we are seeking by adopting principles or constructing theories of justice. Is our aim to minimize the way people interfere with each other, so they can separately pursue their own lives and projects? Is it to maximize the sort of cooperation that allows people to achieve things together that they could never achieve alone? Or is it to create and maintain the best form of life, or the best form of society, independent of the happiness of the individuals in it or its other collective achievements? (Think of the discussions of those questions in Plato's *Republic*.) In the arguments to follow, the focus is mainly on the second of these three questions about the goals of justice: the things we can achieve together that we cannot achieve by ourselves. But the habilitation framework speaks to all three of the questions, as well as some others.

The Plan of the Book and a Short Lexicon for It

Since understanding the book's central aims depends on an initial understanding of some terms that are antiquated (e.g., habilitation) or ambiguous (e.g., health), it will be helpful to address those matters briefly now, along with an equally brief account of the plan of the book.

Habilitation. Some current English dictionaries do not have an entry for "habilitation" at all, and the online *Oxford English Dictionary* now (2011) marks its verb form as obsolete. That is odd, since the term is alive and well in medical contexts and in the ordinary concept of *re*habilitation. There it continues to mean just what the *OED* says it used to mean in general usage: habilitation is "the action of enabling or endowing [a person or thing] with ability or fitness; capacitation, qualification." Here I will often refer to it just as the process of equipping a person or thing with capacities and/or functional abilities, usually as relevant to a given environment.

It is important to keep in mind the diversity of objects that can be habilitated. One can habilitate oneself as well as others, and one's physical and social environment as well as some specific set of people in it. I will make this point repeatedly, but it plays a particularly important role throughout Part Four (Chapters 7–8), where the extent of the parallelism between traits of basic virtue and traits of basic good health is explored at length.

It is equally important to keep in mind three other things. One is that human beings need habilitation and rehabilitation of various forms throughout their whole lifetimes; except intermittently, we are not self-sufficient, nor can we become so. Another is that our need for habilitation is not just equivalent to our need for survival equipment; we need, as well, the equipment to thrive. Without that, we languish, and ultimately put our survival itself at risk. And the third is that much of this habilitation has to be self- provided. We wither, become weak, fail to develop many important abilities, and ultimately fail to thrive if we cannot habilitate ourselves in any important respect, or when everything we need we receive like manna from heaven. These matters will figure in arguments throughout the text, particularly with respect to healthy agency.

Basic justice. As noted earlier, the subject of the book is not the entirety of distributive justice, but rather its most basic part—the area in which plausible theories of justice diverge least, and in fact in large part converge. This part can be described in a number of substantive ways—for instance, by reciting a familiar list of uncontroversial basic goods, rights, or practical possibilities for negotiation among people who hold very different comprehensive theories of justice. Chapter 1 will mention such lists, but there—as well as elsewhere throughout the book—the argument will rely only on the items in such lists that are connected, in a stable way, to a more general, schematic concept of basic justice.

That general concept, addressed in Chapter 1, limits the subject matter of basic justice to those matters of moral concern over which we have some actual control, either through social institutions or individual conduct, and about which we can require things of ourselves and others on grounds we have jointly reasoned out and can practicably enforce.[1] Included in this general concept, by implication at least, are

---

[1] T. M. Scanlon defines the domain of his inquiry in *What We Owe to Each Other* (1998, 6–7), in a similar way, though he declines to identify it with justice. He says it is concerned with the "domain of morality having to do with our duties to other people, including such things as requirements to aid them, and prohibitions against harming, killing, coercion, and deception." But he goes on to say that "[i]t is not clear that this domain has a name . . . [other than, perhaps,] 'the morality of right and wrong.'" He says that the part of morality he has in mind is "broader than justice, which has to do particularly with social institutions. 'Obligation' also picks out a narrower field, mainly of requirements arising from specific actions or undertakings." He thinks the phrase "what we owe to each other" is an apt name for this part of morality and argues throughout his book that this domain "comprises a distinct subject matter, unified by a single manner of reasoning and by a common motivational basis."

the *types* of social norms that generate the rules of "natural" justice (e.g., that similar cases should be treated similarly) and a short list of vaguely described basic goods.

The argumentative strategy of the book will be to explicate that schematic concept of basic justice and notice the way it points toward the need for an elaborate conception of habilitation. Habilitation, in turn, develops into a way of giving the schematic concept of basic justice a more determinate content—one that organizes and clarifies the points of convergence among philosophical theories. These points are argued in Chapters 2–8.

Framing devices. Using any framing device for philosophical argument does several things. For one, it defines the general area of discussion, operating logically as the definition of the universe of discourse. Then, in doing so, it inevitably defines the edges of the discussion, putting some matters close to those edges (or even beyond them) and making others central. Finally, the frame also helps to define a focus—or perhaps, as in a painting or photograph, a set of focal points to which the eye is drawn in sequence. And if the frame is three-dimensional—a framework—it defines the architectural possibilities as well; the sorts of things that can be built upon it.

The framing devices for distributive justice currently in play include at least these: fair agreement for mutual advantage between fully cooperating members of society; the maximization of aggregate welfare, well-being, or opportunity for well-being (within a given society, or in a global context); the pursuit of an ethical ideal in which reason, will, and desire are harmonized; the improvement of social life and individual well-being in genuine communities characterized by shared values, solidarity, and mutual benevolence; the improvement of individual well-being and chances for a good life through the realization of human capabilities or through the protection of individual rights and liberties; the neutralization or correction of disadvantages that are the product of bad luck. One could go on.

It is useful to notice, however, that these framing devices are offered as a defining condition of a *type* of normative theory of justice—or perhaps even of a specific instance of that type—and the whole thing is then put forward against rivals. Criticism then comes from those rivals, or from inside the specific theory, but is typically aimed at dismantling or improving that theory, or type of theory, as a whole.

By contrast, the framing device proposed here is more abstract: that all philosophical inquiry into matters of basic justice should be framed in terms of the concept of habilitation. This is not an effort to replace any specific type of normative theory but rather to recast the framing devices they all use. It is in that sense a meta-theoretic proposal, criticism of which can be separated from criticism of specific types or instances of normative theory. Arguments on these matters appear throughout the book, but most pointedly in Parts One and Two (especially Chapters 2, 4, and 6).

Eudaimonistic health. The habilitation framework gives a central place to "complete" health, defined so as to include physiological and psychological functioning within an environment, on both the negative (e.g., disease) side of the health ledger and its positive (e.g., well-being) side as well. And the resultant focus on health is a focus on what is necessary for each individual, with a particular set of endowments, to develop and sustain various levels of good health in various environments. See especially Chapter 3.

Robustly good (eudaimonistic) health. The definition of good health will be the key to the health scale, and in a nutshell, the definition of robustly good health that will be adopted here is "reliably competent physiological and psychological functioning in a given environment." The so-called negative definition of health, in which health is treated as the absence of pathology, while it naturally receives a good deal of attention in philosophy of medicine and bioethics, is inappropriate here, since it does not adequately cover good health and well-being.

The arguments in Chapters 3–4 and 7–8 develop this focus on robustly good eudaimonistic health in terms of its conceptual connections to ethical theory and contemporary health science. One aim (Chapters 7–8) is to show the extent of the convergence between the norms of basic justice and the motivational structure and behavioral dispositions of the sort of agency characteristic of good health. Another aim (Chapters 4–6) is to show that the focus on this sort of health—and in particular the part of it we may call healthy agency—gives us a currency to use in theories of justice that is equal to or superior to other candidates, such as liberties, entitlements, capabilities, opportunities, well-being, luck, or various combinations thereof.

Representative goods. The notion of a representative good is straightforward. Practical problems are often simplified if we can find a single, observable, and scalable item from which it is possible to infer the presence, absence, quantity, or quality of all the items with which we are concerned. That single item can then become an index for the whole bundle of items we must consider. This is especially important in a theory of distributive justice, where we continually face allocation problems under conditions of scarcity. Answering questions of who should get how much of what there is to distribute depends upon solving—or at least working around—the indexing problem.

Chapters 5–6 concern the definition of an operationalizable health scale, running from worst to best. The definition of the health scale is followed by the proposal that focusing on a particular region on the scale—robustly good health—provides us with a plausible upper boundary for what might be required (as a matter of basic justice) with respect to health. More generally, however, the argument is that health can function as a representative good in normative theories of distributive justice, and that at least for basic justice it is superior, in that role, to various standard alternatives such as wealth and income, subjectively defined welfare or well-being, or preference satisfaction.

Goals and targets. The third proposal of the book is that a particular region of robustly good health—namely, robustly healthy agency—yields an appropriate target for basic distributive justice, even though healthy agency is only one of the goals we have for health, let alone for basic justice itself. It turns out that hitting, or approximating, that target will get us to the other goals as well, with a minimum of wasted effort, since healthy agency is causally connected and approximate to the entire bundle of goals involved. And the healthy agency target is appropriately limited as well, being far from perfect health but even farther from the bottom of the health scale.

The arguments for this proposal are in Chapters 4–6. They are closely entwined, however, with the discussions of agency throughout the book, especially those in Chapters 7–8. They also rely heavily on the landscape of problems framed by the conception of the circumstances of habilitation (Chapter 2), as well as the arguments for eudaimonistic good health as the representative good for justice (Chapter 6).

Rhetorically, these arguments rely on the intriguing relationships between goals and targets—especially in practical circumstances in which outcomes cannot be guaranteed, and thus one must choose strategies rather than outcomes. Consider: even if the archer's only goal is to hit the physical target on the range, the target that the archer will actually choose to aim at will be determined by distance, windage, expected velocity of the arrow, and so forth—and may be quite different from the goal. The archer's actual target will be a virtual one hovering in the vicinity of the actual goal. The argument here is simply that robustly healthy agency covers the other goals well enough that using it as the virtual target will always be sufficient to get to a best approximation to all the goals. The arguments on these matters are found most explicitly in Chapter 6, and throughout Part Four (Chapters 9–10).

Part 1

Habilitation and Basic Justice

Preface to Part One

The two brief chapters in Part One explicate the concepts of basic justice and habilitation (Chapter 1), and the circumstances of habilitation for basic justice (Chapter 2). These preparatory materials are necessary for the arguments of Parts Two, Three, and Four, but they have a supplemental purpose as well. That purpose is to introduce an essential strand of the argument running throughout the rest of the book: namely, that theories of basic justice should be reoriented in a fundamental way—a way that encompasses not only the urgent problems about conflict, cooperation, and coordination under circumstances of scarcity and competing purposes but also encompasses the equally urgent problems about habilitation, health, and the common goals growing out of them.

Typical accounts of basic justice, after all, are implicitly framed by an almost irresistible narrative—human history written as the story of appalling conflict, malice, and resulting injustice, both political and personal. At a political level, this is the story of war and peace, grinding poverty and lavish wealth, slavery and freedom, subjugation and dominance—all of it driven by the struggle for survival in circumstances of scarcity, egoism, fixed loyalties, and the ability of a few to triumph over the many, and to organize their labor. At a personal level, this is the story of fear and greed, hatred and love, cruelty and kindness, selfishness and altruism, and above all, appetites for pleasure and triumph. The emphasis in both stories is on humans who have conflicting primal impulses at war within themselves, and which perpetually threaten to put them at war with each other. The emphasis throughout is on the undeniable, ever present reality of basic injustice.

These chapters emphasize a different aspect of human history. This is a story about the equally undeniable persistence of *basic justice*, along with injustice, and the intimate connection of both to the necessity for human habilitation. It proposes that focusing on the *circumstances of habilitation*—that is, the circumstances under which such habilitation is both necessary and possible—is an appropriate way to understand the circumstances under which basic justice itself is possible, or not. And it proposes that focusing on the circumstances of habilitation leads to making human health—and in particular its agentic powers—central to constructing normative theories of justice.

1

Concepts and Conceptions

Basic Justice and Habilitation

The first task for this chapter is to outline a fundamental part of distributive justice (basic justice) and to persuade readers that it is worthwhile to confine attention to it for the remainder of the book. This is the center of attention in Section 1 below.

Section 2 outlines the concept of habilitation and argues that it is a particularly illuminating tool for examining basic justice. It provides a perspicuous view of the range and nature of those basic problems. It illuminates not only the usual ones but some neglected ones as well.

Section 3 examines two types of normative theory that appear to have especially close conceptual connections to habilitation (capability theories; dependency and care theories). The habilitation framework proposed here is then distinguished from them.

Section 4 suggests that habilitation into a robust form of health is a project central to the human condition itself, rather than to a particular normative theory, and that the habilitation framework could in principle provide a theory-independent framework for normative theories of basic justice generally.

1. Basic Justice

1.1. *General concept and probable content*

For present purposes, let us say that the subject matter of *basic* justice is limited to those matters of moral concern over which we have some actual control, either through social institutions or individual conduct, and about which we can require things of ourselves and others on grounds we have jointly reasoned out, and can practicably enforce.

Notice that this is a very general characterization of basic justice. It does not directly refer to a list of basic goods, duties, prohibitions, liberties, or political mandates—though there are some obvious candidates for such a list. Nor is the term "basic" here derived from a previously defined concept of the basic structure of society. Nonetheless, this general characterization will include by implication a substantial list of formal, procedural, and substantive requirements.

It is not hard to find illustrative examples of such requirements—ones that are firmly and deeply grounded in reasoning that is generally accessible and acceptable to us all. The formal principle that similar cases be treated similarly is almost certainly a part of basic justice in this sense, since it is entailed by formal features of standard logic, and thus ordinary reasoning itself. That formal principle is implicit in the possibility of all rule-making, and it has tempted some writers to treat it as "the" rule of justice (e.g., Perelman, 1967, Ch. II) or as a central element of the procedural principles of "natural" justice.[1] Such elements of natural justice regularly include the principles that people should have advance notice of what they are required to do, in the form of intelligible, determinate, nonarbitrary rules that are possible to follow. By extension, substantive requirements of promise keeping and reciprocity are also, typically, included among the elements of basic justice.

The principles just mentioned could obviously be grouped under the heading of *fairness*. But using "justice as fairness" as a general concept for present purposes is probably not wise; it works better in the context of a particular range of normative theories. Since I want to propose the habilitation framework as something relevant to all normative theories of justice, I want to keep the general concept of its subject matter (basic justice) distinct from any of the developed conceptions of it that particular normative theories might propose. A general concept should be distinguishable from its conceptions.[2]

So for present purposes I want to treat even the formal and procedural principles mentioned earlier as mere illustrative possibilities. The general concept of basic justice will itself remain at the more abstract level given initially, without commitment to a specific content. So, to repeat, it is requirements in general, rather than any specific ones, that are elements of basic justice at this formal level. Among the requirements that might be imposed, the basic ones (in this usage) are those that are practical in a very strong sense: ones that can be justified by reasoning that is accessible (as in philosophy, science, technology, and positive law) to people generally, without regard to their religious or cultural identities; and ones that can be implemented effectively because they concern matters that are at least partially under our control.

---

[1] See the section on Roman law and its procedural version of natural justice in D'Entreves, *Natural Law* (1964); "Eight Ways to Fail to Make Law," from Fuller, *The Morality of Law* (1964); "The Minimum Content of Natural Law," from Hart, *The Concept of Law* (1961, Ch. 9).

[2] The distinction between a general concept and a conception is made with respect to law by Hart, in *The Concept of Law* (1961, 155–59), and later followed with respect to justice by Rawls, *A Theory of Justice* (1971, 5). I employ it primarily with respect to concepts of basic justice, habilitation, and health.

When basic justice in this sense is combined with a full-fledged conception of habilitation (to be developed throughout this book), it will define a substantial agenda for normative theories of justice. It would be disingenuous to suggest that such an agenda will have no framing effects for normative theories. But it will not *necessarily* entail any particular set of substantive, normative principles. To the extent that a given normative theory of justice confines itself to matters of basic justice in the sense used here, and carries out only the agenda defined by the conception of habilitation, it will be, I suppose, a habilitation theory—and so much the better for it, perhaps. But to the extent that a normative theory removes one or another of the limiting criteria of basic justice, or adds to or subtracts from the habilitation agenda, we will simply say that it changes the subject and moves us toward a conception of something else—perhaps comprehensive, complete, perfect, or ideal justice driven by another conception of habilitation or something else.

1.2. *What will be missing*

Ideal justice. A discussion that focuses on basic justice will necessarily exclude some things that attract considerable philosophical attention in other contexts. One of these things is a broad discussion of all the virtues and their connection to each other, and to individual conduct, and to the design of ideal social institutions. We will follow Aristotle (and most subsequent philosophical practice) in excluding this very broad, Platonic agenda from the discussion of justice of a distributive or restorative sort. That does not mean, however, that we will exclude discussions of basic justice as it might itself operate under ideal conditions. Nor does it mean that discussions of aspirational goals connected to basic justice will be shortchanged.

Esoteric reasoning. Discussion-ending appeals to fixed beliefs (secular or religious) whose warrants are esoteric—accessible only to people through their particular cultural or religious or idiosyncratic identities—will be put aside, as previously noted. Their influence as motivational factors will certainly be acknowledged, as will the influence of profound acquired attachments, primal emotional responses, and unconscious drives. Those things will figure importantly in the account of the circumstances of justice. And it may be worth noting here, for people embroiled in debates about the proper place of religious convictions in public affairs, that this bracketing of fixed religious beliefs in no way singles out religious belief. The same bracketing is applied to secular or even purely physiological sources of fixed motivation or belief.

Political realism. A third exclusion is the one represented by Socrates's silencing of Thrasymachus in Plato's *Republic*—namely Thrasymachus's position that justice is not a thing that it is useful to discuss philosophically at all, since it is simply a matter of the strong imposing their will on the weak, or (by extension) a matter of the silencing effect that prejudice, tradition, or conventional social norms can have on all of us. That kind of moral skepticism will not be confronted directly, though its advocates will certainly be addressed by the arguments, with their peculiar use of the term "justice" duly noted. Here the discussion will follow accounts of justice, law, and international relations more complicated than that espoused by Thrasymachus and his successors. It will adopt an all-things-considered account of practical norms (identified with moral norms) grounded in open-source reasoning and justification (Becker, 1973, 364–71; Becker, 1986, Ch. 1). People regularly develop stable, practicable agreements using such norms, even though they disagree dramatically among themselves about more comprehensive normative matters. In that sense it will be a political discussion about basic justice, conducted in terms of public reason in Rawls's sense, though it will not be limited to political liberalism (Rawls, 1999, 131–80).

1.3. *Precedent, historical context, and practical rationale*

The general concept of basic justice adopted here has a long history in practical affairs, and a pedigree in Western philosophy that stretches at least as far back as Aristotle. The pedigree is traced swiftly in Samuel Fleischacker's *A Short History of Distributive Justice* (2006, 1–3). But the history of multicultural empires, governments, legal systems, peacemaking, diplomacy, commerce, exploration, migration, and travel all give evidence of its relevance for practical affairs.

One can make a convincing case that in heterogeneous (and practically urgent) cultural contexts, reflective people interested in pursuing something other than warfare have always employed this concept of basic justice: seeking from each other agreements about requirements whose legitimacy could be established by practical reasoning of a universal sort. After all, an agreement that depends on reasoning that is inaccessible to some of the parties will by definition not be reachable; an agreement that depends on a particular contestable conception of the good (or evil) will either not be reachable or not be stable; an agreement solely about aspirations or ideals rather than requirements will (in many social circumstances) leave many practical problems unsolved; a wholly impractical requirement is aspirational at best, mere hand-waving at worst.

This general concept of basic justice, then, outlines terrain that might be held in common by people who offer a wide assortment of differing comprehensive conceptions of justice (including an amoralist one), but who continue to think that it is possible to work out rational agreements with each other about many of its most fundamental norms. It thus meets the goal of having a general, stipulative concept that fixes ideas for the purpose of productive discussion—and which is as uncontroversial and philosophically innocent as possible.

The temptation to remove the practical constraints on political philosophy. Normative theorists are sometimes impatient with attention to general concepts drawn from practical affairs. The concept of basic justice proposed here, for example, may seem to be a distraction for more purely philosophical purposes. Writers pursuing a normative project within an egalitarian tradition, or a liberal democratic one, or a libertarian one, may be tempted to begin with a general concept of justice that is settled only within their tradition. This is certainly a convenience for like-minded readers, but it carries a risk. Normative theories based on it may lose contact with work in other traditions, or worse, inadvertently misconstrue them as sharing their own general concept of the subject matter.

In particular, though philosophers since Plato have assumed that justice has something to do with fairness, equality, and the impartial application of general rules, it is clear that the meanings of such terms are elastic—historically, culturally, and across contemporary normative traditions.[3] At a theory-independent level, it is probably unwise to lose contact with a concept of equality that emphasizes both the equal treatment of equals and the unequal treatment of unequals, for example, even though in some hands it has been used to endorse slavery, the subordination of women, and the absence of social obligations to help the disadvantaged. Nor is it wise to lose contact with traditions in which a social obligation to help the poor is regarded as a matter of charity rather than justice. Ultimately, since a philosophical theory must be thoroughgoing, it seems wiser to begin it with general concepts that encompass the central elements of both historical and contemporary theories.

---

[3] Samuel Fleischacker, *A Short History of Distributive Justice* (2006), Introduction and Chapter 1, argues persuasively that this has happened with the concept of distributive justice. He says,

> I can hear an objector complaining that people have long believed in human equality and therefore must have implicitly believed in [a notion of equality similar to what one finds in contemporary theories of] distributive justice. People have indeed long believed in human equality. What they have not held is that the equal worth of humanity entails equality in political and social goods—much less in economic goods. . . . The notion that all human beings are in some sense equally deserving of a good life can be found in many societies, across human history. Even Plato justifies his hierarchical republic, in part, by the fact that the hierarchy will be good for those in its bottom echelon. Aristotle similarly says that slavery, when properly conducted, is good for the slaves. Again, Hindu caste hierarchies have been defended by the claim that the suffering that comes with a life at the bottom of the hierarchy will help those who endure their lot uncomplainingly to gain merit by which they can rise to a better life in the next incarnation. But by such arguments it is possible to represent the most inegalitarian society as serving egalitarian ideals. It is an encouraging fact that, as seems to be the case, most cultures have regarded all human beings as equal in some fundamental sense. It is a discouraging fact that this belief does not mean very much as far as equality in social, economic, or political status is concerned. (8–9)

He also makes the point repeatedly through his book that both philosophers and people in religious traditions have tried to reduce the apparent inconsistencies in this history by making a sharp distinction between justice and charity. See, for an overview of some of the contemporary philosophical discussion on this point, Allen Buchanan, "Justice and Charity," *Ethics* 97:3 (1987), 558–75.

The function of a general concept. The point of getting clear about a general concept of basic justice is that we can use it to identify and adjudicate certain fundamental disputes that arise within normative theories and between them. It helps settle questions about whether someone has actually offered a relevant account of the subject at all ("I don't know what you are trying to discuss, but it isn't *basic justice*"), or an incomplete one ("Your account of basic justice covers only a small part of the terrain"), or an inaccurate one ("What you say just doesn't fit the facts"), or an ineffective one ("What you say may be true and on-topic, but how does it help decide anything?"). We can thus expect the general concept of basic justice to establish criteria of relevance, completeness, accuracy, and effectiveness for normative theories of justice.

That is enough, I believe, for this fundamental element of the background to do for present purposes. A schematic concept will suffice, leaving the development of full-fledged conceptions to normative theory.

This is not true of every background element of normative discussions. In some cases we need full conceptions rather than schematic concepts.

2. Habilitation: Concept and Conception

The schematic concept of habilitation will certainly need such further development, since it will define the framework proposed here for philosophical theories of basic distributive justice and will also guide the conceptions of basic health and healthy agency that are central to proposals about the appropriate metric and target for basic justice.

2.1. *General concept, scope, and conception*

General concept. Habilitation, in its central historical sense, is the effort to equip a person or thing with a range of functional abilities or capacities. That is the general concept of it, and it is immediately clear that habilitation in general raises *some* matters of basic justice. Entry-level human beings left entirely to their own devices will not survive, so the practice of providing some habilitation for infants and children is a normatively necessary one for us, conditional only on our prior commitment to preserve their lives, and our ability to do that. Further, human beings of all ages need more than a survival minimum if they are going to thrive—even at a suboptimal level. So some of the questions any normative theory of justice must address will concern how much habilitation should be available *to* whom, and provided *by* whom, and *for* how long.

Scope. It is tempting to think that those questions about habilitation cover only a small part of the territory of distributive justice—perhaps the part that concerns the care of infants and young children, the elderly, and the temporarily or permanently disabled or disadvantaged. But that misses two crucial facts.

The first is that under reasonably favorable circumstances, people who have even a few significant abilities and capabilities go on *to equip themselves* with many additional ones throughout their lives. They habilitate themselves, in ways that generate many of the usual problems of justice having to do with conflict, cooperation, and coordination among fully competent adults.

The second crucial fact is that sustaining the success of all habilitative efforts, whether socially provided or individually achieved, is a process that goes on over the complete lives of individuals in overlapping generations and depends on sustaining a wide array of environmental and social conditions that are either directly or indirectly under our control. Habilitation of all sorts thus generates the usual problems of justice in the design and operation of social institutions and norms.

Attention to those two things makes it clear that questions about habilitation cover the *whole* basket of things required for *all* the abilities or capabilities that are possible for human beings to acquire or sustain, whether through their own efforts or the efforts of others. And one or another of these habilitative possibilities is linked causally to things not only throughout the full range of human possibilities but also to the full range of enabling or disabling social or environmental circumstances in which we might live. As a result, concerns about habilitation ultimately reach all the things implicated in our aspirations and aversions, and which we care enough to strive for, or fight for, or make a claim of justice about.

And habilitation covers even more than justice, if we are using the general concept of basic justice outlined earlier. The subject matter of basic justice is limited to questions about what we can *require* of ourselves and others, and within that, to what can effectively be provided (or made accessible, or attractive) by social arrangements that are effectively enforceable. It is clear, however, that questions about habilitation range over much more than that. For example, we can ask about the extent of the habilitation we would need in order to have some ideal form of human happiness or well-being, or some ideal form of a complete human life.

This more-than-comprehensive coverage of the subject matter of basic justice makes habilitation a good candidate for organizing reflections about it that are independent of particular normative theories. We need not worry that the scope of habilitation is narrower than one or another of those theories, thus making it inadequate as an organizing principle for the whole range of theories.

Habilitation and health. A consequence of focusing on habilitation is that doing so shines an unflattering light on the relative neglect of health in theories of justice. Health is certainly a matter of concern in all of them, in one way or another, but it is not an especially prominent one. There are prominent attempts to apply theories of justice *to* the distribution of health care and to matters of population health.

There are prominent attempts in biomedical ethics to address health research and clinical practice. And there is a prominent connection between health and virtue in the eudaimonistic tradition, as will be discussed in Chapter 3. But in general, *within* standard theories of distributive justice themselves, even ones that focus on well-being or capabilities, health does not have an especially prominent place even among basic goods.[4]

This is startling. After all, it is common to think that good health is the *most* basic thing of all. If we lack it, and cannot get it back, nothing else much matters. When we have it, we have the basis for achieving, enjoying, and making the most of every other basic good. And staying healthy is linked to many of those other basic goods; many of them are necessary for sustaining health. So it is natural to think—almost proverbial to think—that health is at the very center of what matters most to us.

That proverb might of course be misleading. Making health more prominent might have the perverse effect of effacing our legitimate, independent concerns about other matters of justice, such as economic resources, freedom, civil liberties, equality of opportunity, and so forth. Nonetheless, it is hard to think that health should have a *subordinate* place among basic goods. It will turn out in what follows that framing the questions of basic distributive justice as questions about habilitation makes a fundamental place for both physical and psychological health.

3. Normative Theories with a Close Connection to Habilitation

As a further preliminary, it is useful to consider two important currents in contemporary normative theory that are more closely related to habilitation than others. This closeness might raise suspicions about whether the habilitation framework can be genuinely independent of them.

One of these contemporary currents is the capabilities approach to justice. The other is a complex stream of thought that has its origins in concerns about virtue ethics, feminist political theory, gender, the family, dependency, disability, and the ethic of care.

---

[4] Even writers who pursue the so-called medical analogy between virtue and health (e.g., Aristotle; the Stoics) drop the references to health when considering distributive justice, and in general, the paucity of indexed references to health in primary and secondary sources for theories of distributive justice is emblematic of its neglect in those theories. The capabilities approach to justice could easily rectify this. And Martha Nussbaum makes bodily health one of ten categories of central human capabilities. She also alludes indirectly to some elements of mental health (e.g., in the category of emotions), but she does not exploit the opportunity to use it as an organizing principle. See the discussion of the capabilities approach in Section 3 of this chapter.

3.1. *The capabilities approach to justice*

Any framework organized around a conception of habilitation will by definition be a capabilities approach to justice of some sort. Habilitation just *is* about the development of functional abilities, capacities, and capabilities. The question now is about the relationship, if any, between the habilitation framework and the capabilities approach to justice developed by Amartya Sen (e.g.,1985, 2009, and inter alia), Martha Nussbaum (e.g., 2000, 2007, 2011), and other authors as well. It is natural to think that they could be very closely related.

Consider: at one end of a spectrum of possible meanings, an "approach" is every bit as theory-independent as any other framework of background ideas; it might indicate no more than that a particular concept (capabilities) or a particular procedure (social choice theory) will have pride of place in one's inquiries. The argument for such a proposal would consist of showing that orienting things around capabilities is in some way superior to other routes (e.g., those oriented around basic goods, or basic needs) not because it reaches some superior predefined destination, but rather because whatever destination it does reach is likely to be superior, or even optimal.

In fact, my proposal for the habilitation framework does lie somewhere near this minimalist end of the spectrum. So it is a capabilities approach in that attenuated sense, with the caveat that the conception of habilitation developed here, together with the focus on human health and healthy agency, will give considerable structure to this procedure—more structure, in fact, than the originator of the capabilities approach, Amartya Sen, so far endorses.

At the other end of the spectrum, however, taking a capabilities approach might mean defining a full-fledged normative theory of justice rather than a framework—one that is meant to replace other normative theories rather than to reorient them. As I read the authors who have proposed a capabilities approach, they are all closer to the normative-theory end of the spectrum than to the theory-independent framework one.

Amartya Sen's capabilities approach

Amartya Sen's writings on capabilities, which are perhaps the most gently normative on the subject, are nonetheless offered within a firmly egalitarian tradition, and with an emphasis on normative goals of individual freedom and agency defined so as to preserve pluralism about reasons and values at a fundamental level (2009, Chs. 1, 11). Sen also articulates a commitment to developing, via the capabilities approach, what he calls a comparative theory of justice rather than a transcendental one—that is, one whose goal is to remove or ameliorate injustice so as to make the world better than it is, rather than one whose goal is to approximate some transcendental ideal of perfect justice. He argues that a comparative theory of justice can be pursued independently of a transcendental one by beginning with consensus about the nature and existence of various injustices, and then by employing the methods of social choice theory, broadly construed, to find and implement improvements (2009, 3–7, Ch. 4). One then repeats the process indefinitely unless and until consensus about the existence of injustice disappears, to be replaced by loftier and less urgent questions about aspirational matters. This is pretty clearly a normative theory of justice. It is simply defined in terms of an ongoing project with local, recursive processes and comparative aims rather than as a more or less finished blueprint of transcendental principles.

There are, naturally enough, theory-independent elements in Sen's writings on justice, and it is tempting to overemphasize them. After all, Sen often refers to his entire project in meta-theoretical terms—as an "approach" or a "perspective" or an "informational focus" rather than a "specific formula for policy decisions" (2009, 231–33). Nonetheless, his capabilities approach is not theory-independent to the extent proposed here for the habilitation framework, and the two diverge in other important ways as well.

First, Sen's capabilities perspective is, as he says, based on the value of freedom; it is "freedom-based" as opposed to income- or wealth-based, or resource-based (2009, 231). By contrast, the habilitation perspective is based on the objective necessities for human survival, physical and psychological development, and thriving: it is in that sense necessity-based. Whereas Sen emphasizes the fundamental value of freedom (and the correlative importance of agency) throughout human history, habilitation as explicated here will emphasize the objective necessity for developed capabilities throughout every sustained human life and will identify individual health as the most inclusive basic human good in those pursuits. Neither perspective tries to generate a definitive, more or less complete list of the conditions for a good life in terms of some transcendental ideal. But Sen's is driven by a value widely shared by human beings within their lives; the habilitation framework is driven by necessities for human life itself.

Second, as noted, Sen resolutely resists the criticism that his capabilities approach should aim beyond the opportunities opened up by freedom-giving capabilities and instead define a target in terms of actual achievements of some transcendentally defined worthwhile sort. He wants to resist that because he wants to let normative theories and public policies (and the choices made by individuals) emerge from irreducibly plural values by way of comparative forms of reasoning—specifically, reasoning that employs social choice theory, broadly defined. By contrast, the habilitation framework is meant to be suitable for either comparative or transcendental normative reasoning.

Third, although Sen initially offered his capabilities approach as an answer to the question "Equality of what?"—posed as a challenge to Rawls's account of primary goods—it soon developed into something with more sweeping normative consequences. As has been clear since the Dewey lectures in 1984, Sen thinks that by focusing on capabilities (as opposed, for example, to income and wealth, or resources generally) we have a starting point that is closer to our most fundamental concerns about the nature of injustice. Here, the comparison between Sen's capabilities approach and the habilitation framework is perhaps more complex, but the two are no less distinct.

The habilitation framework (as developed throughout this book) will direct us toward structuring our conception of capabilities in terms of healthy human development and will treat such development as fundamentally important with respect to all our concerns about both justice and injustice. It is not clear that Sen would disagree with this, as long as the plurality of reasons and values can be accommodated within the notion of healthy agency. But the habilitation framework will go on to propose health as the representative good for normative theories of justice of all sorts. It is fairly clear that Sen would reject this last move (2009, 231–38).

Martha Nussbaum's capabilities theory

Martha Nussbaum's version of the capabilities approach is more directly normative than Sen's (Sen and Nussbaum, *Quality of Life*, 1993; Nussbaum 2000, 2007, 2011). It employs an objective list of human capabilities that she has developed from a conception of human flourishing drawn from a variety of Aristotelian ethics anchored firmly in modern notions of "the dignity of the human being, and of a life that is worthy of that dignity—a life that has available in it 'truly human functioning,' in the sense . . . of a totality of human life-activities" (Nussbaum, 2007, 74).

From these ethical anchoring points, refined by considering contemporary, cross-cultural notions of human well-being, Nussbaum proposes a list of ten central capabilities as requirements for a life with dignity. They are within the following categories: life; bodily health; bodily integrity; senses, imagination, and thought; emotions; practical reason; affiliation; relation to other species; play; and control over one's environment (Nussbaum, 2007, 76–78).

She describes the capabilities within those categories as "general goals that can be further specified by the society in question as it works on the account of fundamental entitlements which it wishes to endorse. But in some form all are held to be part of a minimum account of social justice: a society that does not guarantee these to all its citizens, at some appropriate threshold level, falls short of being a fully just society" (2007, 75). She goes on to say that she regards her version of the capabilities approach as one version of a human rights approach to basic justice—and one that has the possibility of garnering wide cross-cultural support (2007, 78).

Like Sen's version, Nussbaum's capabilities approach aims to be more general than a set of concrete principles of justice to be applied directly within a given society. Both are offered as open-ended and revisable, sensitive to plural values, and sensitive as well to the aims, resources, and exigencies of various societies in various times and places. Both are firmly in the liberal egalitarian tradition. Unlike Sen, however, Nussbaum is willing to insist on a particular list of human capabilities as general goals for every society and to argue that meeting those goals at some required threshold is essential for basic justice anywhere. That puts her at some distance from Sen's commitment to a comparative approach to justice and brings her into the neighborhood of what he calls a transcendental account of it. Both are normative theories of basic justice, however, and thus sharply distinct from the proposal in this book for a normatively theory-independent habilitation framework for it.

Nonetheless, just as there is a close connection between Sen's emphasis on human agency and the habilitation framework to be offered here, there is also a close connection between Nussbaum's emphasis on human flourishing and the habilitation framework, which itself will be developed from eudaimonistic materials, broadly construed.

It will be wise, as we proceed, to remain aware of these connections. Nussbaum's list of central capabilities has generated considerable philosophical interest, and perhaps a similar amount of interest among philosophically minded social scientists—especially those working in areas of international development and the assessment of it. Keeping this list in mind as we proceed will be a useful test for the habilitation framework. If habilitation is only a framework, and not by itself a normative theory, it should do no more than reorganize and refocus Nussbaum's list. It should not (or not necessarily) eliminate or add items, though it may leave some of them without a direct link to the framework.

Amendments to Sen and Nussbaum

Other philosophers, addressing both Sen's and Nussbaum's capabilities approaches, have offered friendly amendments of a normative sort. In Sen's case, for example, Richard Arneson (1989) and G. A. Cohen (in Sen and Nussbaum, 1993) have argued that it should be taken beyond its normative focus or perspective to press for some specifiable outcomes. Arneson, in particular, thinks of Sen's account as a version of an equal-opportunity-for-well-being thesis.

Jonathan Wolff and Avner de-Shalit's book *Disadvantage* (2007) has addressed Nussbaum's capabilities approach in a similar way—that is, as a version of an equal opportunity thesis. But Wolff and de-Shalit go on to modify Nussbaum's list significantly, partly as a result of reflection on it from a consequentialist point of view, and partly as a result of extensive interviews they conducted with people who have direct experience with the provision of social services in two modern welfare states. Their project will be considered more fully in Chapter 6, Section 6.4. But here it

will suffice to note that their project is avowedly egalitarian, welfarist, and normative. Its empirical part points to a way of gathering evidence, to the standards of
qualitative interviews in social science, for something resembling Nussbaum's list.

The habilitation framework is not another amendment

It invites misunderstanding to consider the habilitation framework as yet another
amendment to the capabilities approach. For one thing, the habilitation framework is more likely to be considered a substitute motion than a friendly amendment—at least by advocates for the capabilities approach. That is partly because
the habilitation framework offers no specific distributive principles or procedures.
As noted in the introduction, it focuses entirely on matters of the metric, currency,
or representative good to be used in a theory of justice. Further, the habilitation
framework proposed here will offer an account of those matters that is decidedly
less pluralistic than those found in current versions of capability theories. So the
arguments of this book will have as much persuasive work to do with capability
theorists as with utilitarians or social contract theorists.

For all those reasons, it seems unnecessarily confusing to describe the framework proposed here as a capabilities approach.

3.2. *Dependency and the ethic of care*

The same is true of theories of justice oriented around notions of dependency and
care. This is another strong current of contemporary social and political philosophy with special relevance to the habilitation framework, but which is distinct
from it. The "care framework" as it might be called emerges from a variety of
sources, in each of which it is part of a more complex body of work. It comes from
virtue theory (especially in its explicitly eudaimonistic versions), feminist political
theory and aspects of both an ethic of care and communitarian theory, as well as
philosophical work on disability and justice. These are, of course, more typically
thought of as separate currents in their own right; they are either distinct normative theories or distinct contributions to others. But each implicitly involves the
general concept of habilitation in a prominent way.

Health, development, and character.[5] Eudaimonistic ethical theory does this by
focusing a good deal of attention on health and human development, emphasizing

---

[5] The relevant philosophical literature on this topic has grown dramatically in the last twenty years.
I mention only a few texts here that are connected in special ways to this habilitation project: Julia
Annas, *The Morality of Happiness* (1993) and *Intelligent Virtue* (2011); Martha Nussbaum, *The Therapy
of Desire* (1994); Margaret Graver, *Stoicism and Emotion* (2007); Paula Gottlieb, *The Virtue of Aristotle's
Ethics* (2009); and three earlier works of my own that are directly involved: *A New Stoicism* (1998a),
"Stoic Emotion" (2004), and "Stoic Children" (1998b).

the extent to which human beings are dependent and underdeveloped at birth and undergo a developmental process over the course of their complete lives that involves what amounts to habilitation at every stage. Moreover, virtue theory of every kind emphasizes the importance, for well-being, of the adequate development, stability and strength of traits of character—traits that amount to capabilities. At the meta-theoretical level, this focus on health, development, and character becomes a more general focus on habilitation designed to develop and sustain those capabilities that are especially important for basic justice, and distinguishing them from capabilities that go far beyond that—capabilities necessary for optimal or ideal levels of well-being, or virtue.

Dependency.[6] Feminist political theory connects with the need for habilitation by focusing on the gendered distribution of labor, especially the labor of providing the care necessary for human health and development during the primary periods of dependency in human life (infancy, childhood, adolescence, and old age). This then leads to important analyses of the gendered aspects of moral psychology, the deeply internalized and institutionalized nature of some basic injustices (found as well in the literature on entrenched disadvantages of all sorts, including critiques of class, race, ethnic, religious, and cultural injustices) and the inadequate responses to such things that are typically found in philosophical theories of justice. Such analyses sometimes lead to explicit criticism of meta-theoretical matters such as the account of the circumstances of justice adopted by a theory of justice.

Community.[7] The same is true of communitarian theory, collectivist theory generally, and work on an ethic of care. All of this work involves a critique of the individualism at least implicitly involved in many classic Western theories of justice. And this work also suggests that renewed attention to the circumstances of justice is called for. Specifically, it suggests that the very concept of a self-sufficient individual human being, independent of mutually supportive human relationships, is of very limited use in normative theory. That concept of self-sufficiency ignores the necessarily social process by which human beings develop into persons and genuine moral agents in the first place, and it ignores the necessarily social circumstances required to sustain healthy human agency. At best, the

---

[6] The literature here is vast and well known for many other reasons as well as the ones singled out here. I mention only the following as the tip of the iceberg: Nancy Chodorow, *The Reproduction of Mothering* (1st ed. 1978; updated edition 1999); Susan Moller Okin, *Gender, Justice, and the Family* (1989); Nel Noddings, *Caring: A Feminine Approach to Ethics and Moral Education* (1st ed. 1984; updated edition 2003); Eva Kittay, *Love's Labor: Essays on Women, Equality, and Dependency* (1998).

[7] I mention, again, only a few works with immediate connections to this project: Michael Sandel, *Liberalism and the Limits of Justice* (1982); Alastair MacIntyre, *After Virtue* (1st ed. 1981; 3rd ed. 2007); Derek Phillips, *Looking Backward: A Critical Appraisal of Communitarian Thought* (1993); Virginia Held, *The Ethics of Care: Personal, Political, Global* (2005); and my "Community, Dominion, and Membership" (1992a).

notion of the self-sufficient individual actor is an abstraction, describing an existence in which human beings can, in special, episodic circumstances, deliberate or act independently of their social circumstances and relationships. At worst, it describes a form of psychopathology. In either case, it is nowhere near complete enough, as a description of human agency, to serve as the basis for a normative theory of justice.

The notion of society or community—without reference to a complex conception of individuality—is also insufficient for normative theory, of course. The description of a society whose basic or perfect justice does not centrally involve the well-being of individuals—individuals who are genuinely individuated—is the description of a dystopic sociopathology.

Interdependence and disability.[8] Philosophical work on disability and justice connects with the need for habilitation (and rehabilitation) through its emphasis on the lifelong interdependence of human beings, their vulnerability to disability throughout their lives, and the analytically distinct components of such disabilities—physiological, psychological, and socially constructed. This then leads to an important emphasis on disabilities, especially disabilities that compromise agency, as a central test case for theories of justice of all sorts.

A focus on habilitation responds directly to this, treating it as a general problem for normative theory. This is obviously not going to be equivalent to the agenda being pursued by philosophical work on disability and justice. Nor should it be, if as I propose, the habilitation framework does not contain specific distributive principles or decision procedures. I think people working on questions of disability and justice may find a focus on habilitation agreeable—as may also be true for people working eudaimonistic virtue theory, feminist ethics, and care ethics. But it will not replace their normative agendas.

4. Habilitation: Conception and Framework

So the focus on habilitation, though it has close conceptual connections to the capabilities approach and theories organized around notions of dependency and care, should be considered quite independent of all of that. Moreover, the argument here will be that we can do better than merely focus on habilitation. Rather, we can develop a particular conception of it that will serve as an organizing framework for

---

[8] See, for example, Anita Silvers, David Wasserman, and Mary B. Mahowald, *Disability, Difference, Discrimination: Perspectives on Justice in Bioethics and Public Policy* (1998); the "Symposium on Disability," *Ethics* 116:1 (October 2005), with contributions from Lawrence Becker, Anita Silvers and Leslie Francis, Jeff McMahon, Eva Kittay, David Wasserman, and N. Ann Davis. See also Nussbaum, *Frontiers of Justice* (2007, Part One).

normative theories of basic justice generally—one that is detailed enough to guide the construction of such theories without substantively prejudicing them.

The following chapters provide that development, first through an account of the circumstances of justice (as seen through the lens of habilitation), and then through an account of the connections between basic justice and habilitation into health, broadly defined, and with particular reference to healthy agency. But it may be worth closing this chapter by addressing, in a preliminary way, a question that is likely to be in the background for many readers throughout the book.

Why habilitation, again? At the level of general concepts, all the following have important similarities: habilitation, dependency, interdependency, community, disability, and care. They can all be used, to varying extents, as organizing concepts for particular normative theories of justice. The same can be said about fairness, mutual advantage, well-being, virtue or excellence, and merit.

Among them, however, this book will argue that habilitation is the more inclusive organizing concept. It can frame an investigation into all the others, but the reverse is not the case.

Consider capabilities. As this approach to justice has been developed, it has focused on the capabilities of individual human beings, and some of its advocates treat it as similar to a human rights theory. This will make it awkward to give direct attention to two of the three dimensions of habilitation: habilitating the physical environment, and doing the same for the social environment. Opportunities, freedom, well-being, human excellence, and merit have the same difficulty. Fairness and mutual advantage are similar and also have the disadvantage of containing something very like a particular distributive rule.

Or consider various forms of an ethic of care. They focus on a relationship, *caring-for* another, that depends upon but is distinct from *caring-about* another. In a caring-for relationship, there are givers and receivers, and the givers care about the well-being of the receivers. These relationships are often reciprocal, and they are always personal, at least at the level of the giver's moral imagination and motivation.

Care is thus too narrow to be an organizing principle for normative theories of basic distributive justice generally. Some of the most pointed concerns in the area of basic justice are about situations in which caring relationships do not and perhaps cannot arise. Some major theories of distributive justice address these very situations in ways antithetical to a primary emphasis on caring relationships (think of utilitarian and mutual advantage theories). So proposing care as an organizing principle for theories generally will hardly be theory-independent. It will remain a competing form of normative theory.

Habilitation, by contrast, covers both caring relationships and ones in which people are mutually disinterested. It covers both personal relationships and decidedly impersonal ones. It is about equipping ourselves and others with anything we might need in order to function in our environments. This typically includes care, but not necessarily so, in some extreme environments. (It seemed to the anthropologist Colin Turnbull to have been virtually extinguished among the Ik people in mountainous Uganda, when he did two years of fieldwork with them. See Turnbull, *The Mountain People,* 1972. Touchstone edition, 1987.) And it includes, by definition, every other good that might be a matter of basic justice as well. Thus it is maximally inclusive of basic goods of concern in normative theories of basic distributive justice and a plausible candidate for a theory-independent organizing framework for such theories. The same cannot be said for care.

I shall argue throughout the book that for similar reasons, the habilitation framework for normative theories of basic justice is the best available one. My aim here is to ensure that this framework and the target projected from it (healthy agency) have an important role to play in every such normative theory.

2

The Circumstances of
Habilitation for Basic Justice

Since habilitation is being proposed here as a framework for theories of basic justice, the proposal should pay some explicit attention to the circumstances under which habilitation is both possible and necessary. As it turns out, this effort will, in effect, enlarge and revise various versions of the account of the "circumstances of justice" currently in use. And it will effectively replace them with this: *The circumstances of habilitation for basic justice are those under which hospitable social environments can arise and be sustained.*

The argument for this will proceed by comparing some traditional accounts of the circumstances of justice to those suggested by the habilitation framework (Section 1), then describing in more detail the circumstances of habilitation (Section 2). Those results will then be summarized (Section 3) and the connection to health duly noted (Section 4).

1. Humean Accounts

In Hume's now classic usage, the circumstances of justice are those features of the human condition that make the acquired virtue of justice—that is, the construction, internalization, and use of its norms—both possible and necessary. He lists a quartet of circumstances: limited altruism, moderate scarcity, rough equality of power, and rough equality of vulnerability (*Treatise,* bk 3.2.2; *Enquiry,* pt 1.3).

In *A Theory of Justice,* Rawls incorporates Hume's list into one aimed at describing the subjective and objective circumstances in which human *cooperation* is both possible and necessary (1971, 126–31). That is probably an enlargement of Hume's overall frame of reference as well as an enlargement of his list. Though Rawls says that his summary of the circumstances of justice "adds nothing essential to [Hume's] much fuller discussion" (128), he mentions some additional things of special relevance to his own theory—such as that the parties care about the well-being of some people in succeeding generations, and that they have different ends, or conceptions of the good life which lead to competing claims. And he makes a point of mentioning in passing some important points about "various shortcomings of knowledge, thought, and judgment" which have consequences relevant to theorizing about justice (127).

As many commentators have pointed out, however, both Hume and Rawls seem preoccupied with resolving conflicts between self-interested individuals who are, at bottom, acting independently. People may be acting in a social setting dense with cooperative norms; they may have attachments to others and interests in others' welfare for its own sake. But the background theory-building assumption is that the fundamental problems of justice somehow lie underneath existing social necessities and norms, in the struggle between self-interest and mutual interest, and between individual interests of any kind (selfish or not) and the a priori demands of justice.

If such underlying struggles are the most fundamental ones, as many political philosophers have taken them to be,[1] then it does seem plausible to define the circumstances of justice in a way similar to Hume's. The question is whether that statement of the fundamental problems is adequate.

It is not adequate for the habilitation framework. For one thing, it is not elaborate enough to deal with the large range of cases in which problems of justice arise for people who already share strong social norms for cooperative behavior and a sharp sense of the injustice of acting against such norms. These people do not always have strongly motivated forms of self-interest; they do not always have sharply distinct, autonomous forms of agency operating independently of shared social norms. (Think of people whose lives are permeated by intense attachments to familial, tribal, ethnic, class or caste, religious, sexual, or national identities which subordinate "merely selfish" interests.) Those people have conflicts about justice, of course, but not necessarily conflicts traceable to the struggle between personal self-interest and the norms of justice—or to conflicts traceable to scarcity or inequality of power and vulnerability. Rather, those conflicts are often about the interpretation of membership in the group, the priorities within it, the distributive consequences of those priorities, and the changes that need to be made in existing social norms in order to improve them. The items on Hume's list figure into this only indirectly, or weakly. In those cases, Humean circumstances remain relevant but not comprehensive.

---

[1] Begin with Plato's *Republic*, Book II; substitute sin for self-interest to get a similar account in many theological accounts of justice; consider state of nature thought experiments, from Hobbes's *Leviathan* onward. Rawls emphasizes this aspect of the circumstances of justice by focusing on the ways in which people can be thought of as mutually disinterested, not because they are exclusively self-interested but because their interests are "the interests of a self that regards its conception of the good as worthy of recognition and that advances claims in its behalf as deserving satisfaction" (*A Theory of Justice*, 1971, 127).

Focusing on habilitation, since it concerns equipping ourselves and others with the functional abilities we need to survive and thrive, is likely to lead to a more comprehensive account of the circumstances of justice. It is hard to think of cases which would escape such an account. If there is no damage to functional abilities—or risk or threat of such damage—there is presumably no basic injustice, even though the situation or events in question might be far from ideal. But since the subject here is basic justice, rather than ideal justice, if we give an account of the circumstances under which we can and cannot equip ourselves and others with functional abilities we will likely have captured the full range of circumstances in which problems of basic justice arise.

In any case, since habilitation is offered here as a covering concept for theorizing about basic justice, it will need a conception of the circumstances under which habilitation can be accomplished. For the reasons just mentioned, I will treat that task as equivalent to developing a conception of the circumstances of basic justice. In what follows, when it seems important to do so, I will remind readers that I am speaking of the circumstances of justice in this special habilitative sense—the one that gives this chapter its title. Otherwise, I will elide the full phrase either to *circumstances of habilitation* or to *circumstances of justice*, as seems appropriate in the context.

2. Functional Abilities in a Given Range of Environments

The most fundamental and general circumstances of habilitation have to do with the most fundamental and general facts about our humanness and our need for habilitation. This section surveys such factors and the habilitative tasks they generate for human beings. The concluding section condenses and summarizes the circumstances of habilitation, and indicates the way in which all of them point toward the importance of human health and healthy agency. The chapters of Part Three of the book will return to these matters in more detail.

The factors of habilitation come from features of our physical and social environments and features of our individual physical and psychological endowments. Some of these define necessities for habilitation and others define its possibilities. When necessities are met by impossibilities and it is within our control to make the impossible possible, there are some obvious connections between habilitation and basic justice.

The environmental, social, and personal dimensions of habilitation. Whether we get the habilitation we need at each stage of our development, and continuously throughout our lives, depends upon the fit between our environments and our physical and psychological abilities. That is, it depends upon the availability of necessary resources to people with our physical and psychological abilities, even when those resources are plentiful in the physical and social environment. (Without the necessary physical and psychological abilities to acquire and use resources, we suffocate or die of exposure or starve before we can equip ourselves or be equipped to survive.) But it depends equally on the way those resources are distributed throughout the environment. (Starvation is often a distributive problem rather than one of absolute scarcity.) And when resources are or threaten to become functionally unavailable or maldistributed, we face a rehabilitative problem: one of restoring an adequate fit between those resource problems and the personal abilities—agentic and cooperative—in the people within our environment.

Three habilitative tasks. In general terms, we all face three distinct habilitative tasks in any environment: (1) acquiring and sustaining the functional abilities necessary and sufficient for our own well-being, through our own efforts and the efforts of others; (2) helping others to acquire such functional abilities, through their own efforts and our help, as necessary; and (3) helping to habilitate the physical and social environment where necessary—for example, by making its resources available to people with our functional physical and psychological abilities.

2.1. *Circumstances in which habilitation is necessary*

State of nature stories. A state of nature thought experiment for the habilitation framework will be a very short one for solitary humans who lack adequate survival abilities. That will be true in any physical environment for infants, young children, and anyone else who lacks the agentic powers (physical or psychological) to survive without the help of others. Habilitation precedes survival abilities.

The same is true for groups of humans which cannot produce survival abilities in enough of their members to become self-sustaining. Such groups will lack either the social norms or distribution of agentic powers within the population to provide adequate survival assistance for the group itself and those within it—in whatever range of physical environments and/or changed social environments may be accessible to them. For all such human beings, solitary individuals and groups, adequate habilitation for survival will be impossible, and however rich in resources their physical environments may be, their situations will be lethal. Often immediately.

Survivors. A brief survival story is possible for solitary individuals who are already sufficiently habilitated to live on their own for lengthy periods. They will have to have appropriate agentic strength and power of a survival sort, including initiative, endurance, perseverance, and adaptability, when they are thrust into their solitary state. Even so, survivor stories will be short ones unless at least one of the physical and social environments accessible to them is minimally hospitable. If not, the threats to their survival from harsh physical conditions and hostile neighbors will be continuous, urgent, and debilitating. Their lives will be genuinely Hobbesian: solitary, poor, nasty, brutish, and short.

The same is true for radically unorganized groups of individuals—ones which lack the social norms and distribution of agentic powers among their members necessary for long-term, multigenerational survival. They do not have a lengthy survival story either. And the story that they do have will also likely be almost Hobbesian: not necessarily solitary, and perhaps not poor or nasty or brutish, but certainly short in some environments.

It is important to notice, however, that the cause of their truncated lives need not involve a Hobbesian war of each against all. Groups can simply collapse of their own weight, or be overwhelmed by human or animal predators, or epidemic diseases, or natural disasters. The historical and anthropological record does not support the notion that such collapses always involve an internal war of each against all—even in cases of extreme scarcity in the physical environment. (Think of slave labor camps, or even death camps.) Rather, such groups may simply disintegrate, or if unconfined, simply scatter—either permanently or until the immediate threat recedes. Nonetheless, if the group lacks the distribution of agentic skills among its members necessary to respond to threats to its existence, its life will also be genuinely Hobbesian in result.

Primal survival groups. For the habilitation framework, state of nature stories all begin with social groups structured for multigenerational survival. It is only in those social situations in which human beings can be born and habilitated well enough to survive, reproduce themselves, and sustain the sort of minimally hospitable social environment for long enough for that to happen. And a necessary feature of the social structure of such a group will be the social practices and/or norms which sustain habilitative behavior sufficient for successful reproduction.

Without the emergence of these primal survival groups, the evolutionary track leading to our hominid precursors would have been extinguished long before something approximating our current mammalian form emerged. No doubt these precursor groups of our distant non-mammalian ancestors were merely instinctively social to the necessary extent; what we call intentional behavior in accordance with social norms did not exist. But we can easily imagine how, once consciousness and intentional behavior evolve, social norms underwriting survival instincts might also arise. In fact, in the typical course of human development they would have to rise if for no other reason than to resolve situations in which conflicting instinctive motivations are in equipoise and pose a conscious decision problem. Decision procedures emerge from repeated decision problems like that, and become habitual. Conflicting personal habits generate coordination problems which social norms resolve. So it is plausible to think that they evolve along with the earliest emergence of primal survival groups, rather than subsequently.

But these precursors to the primal survival group states of nature are not the ones relevant to the habilitation framework being discussed here—except insofar as they might have left traces in our physiological and psychological endowments. What we want to begin with are the primal groups whose survival and reproductive behavior are motivated not only by instinct but also by the recognition of the habilitative necessities for human survival, and by social norms prompted by those instincts and that recognition. At that point we have one of the circumstances of habilitation for justice. (Prior to it, we have only a circumstance for group survival.)

Failure to survive. Even with a behavioral and normative structure suited for survival in their environments, some of these groups will fail to survive, of course. Some will succumb to lethal challenges posed by their physical and social environments, despite their best efforts (fatigue, failure to protect the group or to defend it against external aggressors, or the inability to adapt to novel necessities). Others will fail to make their best efforts and will fail from self-inflicted ventures (self-destructive wars, for example, or ill-advised treaties with warlike neighbors, or the maltreatment of large sections of their own population that then leads to implosion).

Failure to thrive. An indirect cause of the failure to survive, both for individuals and for groups, is the failure to thrive. This is sometimes traceable to deficiencies in individual endowments, physical or psychological. But it is also traceable to environmental factors: to the lack of a physical and social environment within which a self-sustaining multigenerational population can not only survive but thrive.

Guaranteeing merely a survival minimum for human beings turns out to be insufficient to support sustained development (or even sustained survival) for them. Infants tend to decline relative to their peers if they fail to thrive. Failure to thrive can come from poor nutrition (even when it is adequate for survival), physical disease or injury, and environmental factors including physical or emotional neglect and abuse. The predictable consequences of prolonged failure to thrive include permanent deficits in the rate and extent of physical, intellectual, emotional, and social development throughout life. And such deficits are predictably correlated with a wide range of factors that reduce life expectancy. They are thus also predictably correlated with the decline and ultimate disintegration of social groups.

The circumstances of habilitation thus include the circumstances under which human beings can thrive. Defining those circumstances takes us directly to the matters considered in Part Two of this book: the nature of the sort of physical and psychological health relevant to habilitation, as well as the nature of the requisite form of agency.

Developing and sustaining hospitable environments. The environmental dimension of the ability to thrive yields a related circumstance of habilitation: the necessity for developing and sustaining what we may call a genuinely hospitable social environment—one which can generate a self-sustaining, multigenerational core of thriving individuals.

This has consequences for the habilitation of physical environments as well as social ones, and individuals as well as social groups. It will obviously require developing the social norms within the group that are sufficient for habilitating and sustaining both the population itself and the social environment. It will require finding, or developing, a physical environment in which this can occur. And it will require extensive habilitation for at least some individuals' well-being. All these matters have a direct connection to both health and basic justice. They will be considered at length in Part Three of the book.

So to summarize: the state of nature story reveals a complex developmental necessity for habilitation—a direction for both social and physical environments that runs from mere survivability to genuine hospitability, and a direction for (at least some) individuals that runs from survival to the functional physiological and psychological abilities needed for thriving.

2.2. *Circumstances in which habilitation is possible*

It is obvious from the historical and anthropological record that there have been, and still are, many genuinely hospitable social environments—many such environments, that is, for a more or less self-sustaining elite portion of the population. But these long-lasting social environments can apparently occur in the form of a slave society, or a caste society, or one in which half the population is subordinated to the tasks of childbearing and caregiving (to the detriment of their health and life expectancy), and a large percentage of the other half is subordinated to similarly dangerous and unhealthy tasks: hard physical labor in mines, on farms, in construction; in fighting wars.

The connection to basic justice starts to become more obvious when we consider the possibilities for habilitation rather than its necessities. The possibilities have to be in place before the necessities can be met. A substantial part of the argument of this book (Part Two) will be that health is the centerpiece of these possibilities for habilitation, and that healthy agency is the crucial factor in meeting habilitative necessities. It will then turn out that the behavioral and motivational traits of healthy agency will parallel the norms of basic justice quite closely (Part Three).

Remarks about these matters here will be quite brief. Some relevant details will be added as the argument proceeds, but for the moment consider these three general categories of such possibilities for habilitation: the possibility of migration to new environments; the possibility of transforming a given environment through human agency; and the functional abilities of the human agents within them.

Habilitative migration. When a given physical or social environment makes further habilitation impossible or difficult, it may be possible for individuals or whole groups to meet their habilitative necessities through migration. There are many reasons for migration, of course, but the possibility of doing so for habilitative reasons is the one at issue here.

Assume, for the moment, that there is an alternative physical and/or social environment which is more favorable for habilitation than the one now occupied by a given individual or group. The question then becomes one of the accessibility of that alternative environment. That question has two parts: the possibility of emigration and the possibility of immigration. If the migrants cannot get to the new environment soon enough, or adapt to it quickly enough, or fully enough, to access its advantages, migration will fail from a habilitative standpoint. The historical record is replete with details about how these things work out, or fail to work out—both for the migrants and for the places and people on the receiving end, not to mention those left behind. And the connections to questions of basic justice are obvious.

Moderately malleable physical and social environments: stability and control. An alternative to migration is the possibility that the existing physical or social environment can be changed, through human activities, to make it more favorable for habilitative development. This is a fundamental circumstance of habilitation for basic justice.

Let us say that a physical or social environment is malleable to the extent that, through human activities, it can be controlled so as to make it either more or less hospitable. And let us say that a physical or social environment is stable to the extent that it cannot be so controlled.

Both perfect stability and perfect control are problematic for habilitation. Perfect stability means no control through human agency; what we have, or what is ineluctably given to us, is what we are stuck with. Perfect control, however, means no stability; everything requires constant attention because everything that happens is a product of what we do. In neither case are we likely to be able to satisfy the necessities for habilitation.

So the relevant circumstance of habilitation is moderate malleability in our physical and social environments—the area between the extremes of perfect stability and perfect control that makes habilitation of our environments possible, given the functional physical and psychological abilities we have (either individually or collectively).

Health and agency. Ultimately, what makes habilitation possible is in large part the functional abilities brought to it by those involved in habilitative activities. And this brings us to matters of health and agency.

Meeting the habilitative necessities in a given physical environment includes creating and sustaining a genuinely hospitable social environment. And in every case that task will require a population of physically healthy, strong and resilient agents capable of independent work as well as effective cooperative work. This will require substantial psychological health as well, of the sort that supplies agentic initiative and energy (rather than inanition), and the sorts of sociability that make effective cooperative work possible (conviviality—that is, pleasure in living with others; sympathetic understanding of others' habilitative needs; and a willingness to participate in the level of mutual restraint and mutual aid necessary to sustain social life).

The details of such physiological and psychological health will be explored in later chapters. Here it is important only to observe that these details will vary considerably from individual to individual depending on their physiological and psychological endowments and hence their capacity for developing, through habilitation, the functional agentic abilities needed. Typical human agentic endowments include primal and persistent impulses toward a long list of fundamental things: self-preservation, need satisfaction, the pursuit of self-defined goals, reciprocal interactions with others, the recognition of others' similar impulses, impulses to coordinate conduct with others, to acquire communicative abilities (signals; language), to acquire the empathy to understand others, and the seeds of practical reasoning and even strategic thinking. (Infant food-seeking behavior typically exhibits much of this inventory of impulses quite early.) All of this helps to develop the forms of mutuality that make social coordination, cooperation, and conflict resolution possible.

However, along with these primal impulses which contribute directly to the development of prosocial agentic behavior, there are others which complicate agentic action in a social context: primal fight or flight responses, for example; and emotional responses of a disconnective kind, including those such as fear, anger, envy, resentment, biases, and fixed commitments and attachments.

Healthy human development will include the development of all of these primal impulses, even in people who for other reasons already turn out to be assets rather than enemies of a genuinely hospitable social environment. The subsequent variety of personalities will be wide enough to be challenging for the possibilities and necessities of continuing habilitation.

And those possibilities and necessities themselves will be quite varied given the variety of living conditions in potentially or genuinely hospitable social environments. In challenging physical environments, for small-scale, isolated, hunter-gatherer social groups, there will be a premium on physical fitness and resilience for both children and adults. Memory and communicative abilities will be highly prized, but a written language may not be. Literacy may be like magic, available only to a few. Serious illness or injury is likely to be a death sentence. That is a sharp contrast to the range of physical and psychological health and ill health compatible with habilitation for large-scale industrialized social environments with a highly articulated division of labor.

The important point here, in this general statement about habilitative necessities and possibilities, is simply that a level of health and agency appropriate to the physical and social environment is one of the circumstances of habilitation, in all survivable environments.

Mutual advantage and reciprocity. Health at a level that makes a genuinely hospitable social environment possible has consequences for social structure. Healthy agents are strong, resilient, active, and effective agents capable of acting independently. That means they have their own goals, and plans for achieving them. That means they have some competence in making and carrying out the plans necessary for achieving them. They may be convivial, and sympathetic to others' needs. But they will also be self-centered—concerned with pursuits they define for themselves. They will, as Rawls puts it in his account of the circumstances of justice, want to have their own ends recognized as worthy of respect. And for some people, this self-centeredness will have the most prominent role in their motivations—whether they are acting on their own behalf or on behalf of others.

This obviously leads to both internal conflict (self-centeredness versus other centeredness) and interpersonal conflict. Resolving such conflicts in a reliable way is important for habilitation: one of the things that makes cooperation possible, and thus makes meeting habilitative necessities possible.

Reliable patterns of behavior with respect to cooperation, coordination, and conflict resolution—whether in the form of individual behavioral traits independent of social norms, or traits filtered through and reinforced by strong social norms—help to resolve conflicts and thus to make cooperation possible and reliable. And there are two especially important social norms that are almost immediately available to psychologically healthy agents from early childhood onward. One of these is based on the awareness of the option of mutual advantage as a solution to conflict. Another is based on the awareness of the power of reciprocal behavior in managing cooperative behavior. The way such awareness emerges from healthy human development will be addressed in subsequent chapters. The important general points here are simply the following.

Mutual advantage allows all the involved individuals to be both self-centered and cooperative. If cooperation offers something for everyone involved—and in fact in terms of habilitation usually offers more for everyone than noncooperative behavior—it is a very powerful solution to conflict. It obviously does not solve every conflict, since sometimes the risks involved in cooperative behavior will result in uneven sacrifices across the population (e.g., the way risks are unevenly loaded onto the young for childbearing and war fighting). But a social norm that encourages conduct for mutual advantage seems available across the whole range of possible social environments.

Reciprocity reinforces and extends a norm of mutual advantage. It reinforces mutual advantage by adding agentic control over situations in which acting for mutual advantage is either futile or directly damaging. (I will cooperate if others do likewise, but not otherwise.) Thus a norm of reciprocity makes cooperation conditional for each agent on the similar conduct of others—enough others to make the cooperative conduct effective. And as an empirical matter, norms of reciprocity regularly also make cooperation conditional on proportional benefits and burdens.

Reliable patterns of cooperative behavior make meeting habilitative necessities possible. And that typically means patterns of social behavior involving cooperative conduct for mutual advantage, regulated by social norms of reciprocity.

3. Summary of the Circumstances of Habilitation

The subject of basic justice directs our attention to practical possibilities. The habilitation framework focuses on practical possibilities that are habilitative. Human habilitation requires hospitable social environments. So the preceding discussion of the necessities and possibilities for habilitation can yield the following single-item definition of the circumstances of habilitation

The circumstances of habilitation for basic justice are those under which hospitable social environments can arise and be sustained.

Such compression has its uses, and is harmless as long as it directs attention to a fuller account. The central elements of such a fuller account will include the items discussed in Section 2 of this chapter. Some of those, in turn, will be elaborated considerably in Parts Two and Three of the book.

4. The Centrality of Health and Agency

There is no distributive rule in all of this other than what is implicit in the distribution of agentic powers necessary for creating or sustaining a genuinely hospitable social environment, given its scale, form of social organization, exit options, existing social norms, and the hostile or hospitable nature of the accessible physical and social environment surrounding it. But it is clear that the requisite level of human health—and particularly agentic health—will be central to circumstances of habilitation in every environment.

Part Two of the book, following immediately, describes the requisite conception of human health and argues that the metric of such health can serve as a representative good in theories of basic justice generally (no matter what their distributive principles or rules may be). And it argues that agentic health—robustly healthy agency, as I will call it—can serve as an appropriate target for basic justice.

Part 2

Health, Healthy Agency, and the Health Metric

Preface to Part Two

The following four chapters give an account of the conception of health and the health metric proposed for the habilitation framework. Some aspects of the connection of these matters to basic justice, and their adequacy as a metric for it, will be pursued further in Parts Three and Four of the book. But this Part presents the essentials.

Chapter 3 develops the notion of eudaimonistic health—a conception of physiological and psychological *good* health as well as bad health. This conception of health, while similar to a much criticized definition offered by the World Health Organization (WHO), is distinct from it and avoids the usual objections to the WHO definition. Recent psychological and philosophical work on happiness and well-being is also consistent with the notion of eudaimonistic health developed here.

Chapter 4 refines the notion of eudaimonistic health further by developing the central notion of *basic* good health as *reliably competent physical and psychological functioning in a given environment*. Habilitative abilities, coping abilities, and agency are all in turn central to competent functioning. And the account of basic good health, as distinct from ideal or perfect health, promises to be useful for the limited normative principles of basic justice.

Chapter 5 develops a health scale, or metric, ranging from worst to robustly good basic health, an adequate marker of which lies in healthy agentic powers. This is an obvious target for habilitation of the sort required by basic justice.

Chapter 6 argues that healthy agency can be used as the representative good for basic justice, replacing income and wealth, and pluralistic accounts of basic goods.

3

Eudaimonistic Health

Complete Health, Moral Development, Well-Being, and Happiness

The habilitation framework requires the adoption of a notion of "complete" health—that is, a unified conception of good and bad health, along both physical and psychological dimensions, in a given physical and social environment. Sections 1 and 2 make that case, and note its connection to eudaimonistic ethical theory.

Sections 3 and 4 propose a way of intertwining the notions of health, moral development, well-being, virtue, and purely psychological happiness in the habilitation framework. They reiterate that this intertwining is eudaimonistic in spirit but does not actually amount to a commitment to eudaimonistic normative theory. And they show that this conception of complete health is consonant with recent psychological and philosophical work on positive health and happiness.

Some additional introductory remarks to this chapter may be helpful.

The habilitation framework and its connection to health. As frequently noted by political philosophers in recent years, many historic discussions of distributive justice have begun by addressing a population of healthy, fully functioning adults—or adult males—postponing discussions of the family, and of children, and of the chronically ill or disabled, until the general outlines of the theory are settled. With respect to fully functioning adults, it then seems unremarkable to treat health as one thing in a list of instrumental goods. This initial focus on healthy adults, and the postponement of questions about others, seems to occur at the pretheoretical stage. It is a decision made in the background, before the real theoretical work gets started.

This pretheoretical choice has unfortunate results. Once the postponed questions are eventually addressed, we find ourselves in the middle of contentious debates about how much "we" can reasonably be expected to do around the margins for those who are disadvantaged by gender roles, caring for children, disabilities, or caring for the elderly and disabled. This has been pointed out by many writers, including Okin (1989) and Kittay (1998). Nonetheless, by the time this is pointed out we may be so attached to the theory we have worked out that it is hard to see the need for fundamental change.

By contrast, the habilitation framework focuses attention on all human beings throughout the course of their whole lives, framing every discussion about basic justice in a way that treats health as a primary good, and chronic disadvantages associated with it as an indication that something connected to justice may have gone badly wrong. And health, once it is framed in terms of questions about habilitation, turns out to be a capacious, multidimensional region of many functional abilities, with orderly causal connections to each other.

Healthy agency appears to lie at the intersection of all these abilities, much in the way that eudaimonistic conceptions of health and virtue suppose it is. This raises the intriguing possibility that a conception of health drawn from the eudaimonistic tradition might unify the negative and positive sides of the ledger—directly addressing all the basic elements of well-being as well as health in a medical sense. It will be even more intriguing if it also provides a clear, limiting boundary between the level of good health central to normative theories of justice (particularly basic justice) and perennially contentious conceptions of the good life. Such a conception of health would further define possibilities and necessities for habilitation that are matters of concern for any normative theory of justice.

1. Health, Well-being, and Virtue

In ancient Greek ethics of a eudaimonistic sort, habilitation into health was understood as a part of habilitation into ethical life generally. In those theories, the final end is understood to be one or another form of human flourishing, and progress toward that end is understood to track healthy human development—especially psychological development—for a substantial stretch. This is so because both psychological health and human excellence in general require the same initial assortment of emotional, intellectual, and conative traits, all of which are assumed to rest on some basic physical traits.[1] At some point, once a robust form of physical and

---

[1] See "Philosophy and Medicine in Antiquity," in Michael Frede, *Essays in Ancient Philosophy* (1987). Martha Nussbaum emphasizes the medical analogy throughout *The Therapy of Desire,* but especially in Chapters 1–2. See also Paula Gottlieb, *The Virtue of Aristotle's Ethics* (1994, Ch.1, 20 ff.) in which she argues that Aristotle's use of a medical analogy to introduce his doctrine of the mean (*Nicomachean Ethics* II 1104a12–18) should be taken very seriously. It provides evidence for the view that, like health, ethical virtue has a great deal to do with equilibrium—what I will often refer to later as homeostatic functioning. Virtue as "the mean," she argues (22–25), should not be understood in terms of moderation but rather in terms of equilibrium.

psychological health has developed in early adulthood, what is necessary for further development toward virtue may go well beyond health in that conventional sense. But in the eudaimonistic tradition, to be a healthy adult is by itself to be equipped with at least rudimentary forms of the traits we call virtues when they are more fully developed: courage, persistence, endurance, self-command, practical wisdom, and so forth.

This congruence between health and virtue comes in some measure from the fact that eudaimonistic theories have a wider conception of health than many of us now use, at least in health policy contexts. Ancient Greek eudaimonists do not make a sharp distinction between psychological health and well-being, or between health defined negatively (as the absence of disease, deficit, or injury) and health defined positively (as the presence of stable, strong, and self-regulating traits that contribute to something more than mere survival). In fact, the Stoics (at least some of them, sometimes) appear to run the analogy between health and virtue all the way to a common vanishing point, and to think of perfect virtue as perfect health (Becker, 1998, Ch. 6 and its Commentary).

This analogy between health and virtue is not as alarming as it may sound in the present context. For present purposes, the general concept of basic justice is limited to practicable, enforceable requirements. Perfect health and perfect virtue are quite evidently beyond those limits. But that is something the eudaimonistic tradition clearly acknowledges. Perfect virtue is found only in sages, whose existence is rare if not mythical. The level of health and virtue that even the most diligent, wise, and fortunate people regularly reach is well below the ideal. Except for the most strenuous Stoics, eudaimonists find much to admire and praise in such ordinary levels of virtue. And more to the point here, there is no evidence that even Stoics support enforceable *requirements*, as a matter of justice, to bring themselves and their students from robust health to something approximating perfection. Nor do they think that someone's failing to be a sage calls for medical intervention. Unless this point is understood, however, a eudaimonistic conception of health can be troublesome in a contemporary context.

1.1. *The World Health Organization's definition of health*

Consider the persistent debate about the World Health Organization's definition of health, which appears in the Preamble to its Constitution and seems to be drawn from the eudaimonistic tradition. The definition is given in the first of the nine principles about health that are said to be "basic to the happiness, harmonious relations and security of all peoples" (World Health Organization, 2011). The second and sixth principles explicate the definition more or less directly.

The first principle defines health as "a state of complete physical, mental, and social well-being and not merely the absence of disease or infirmity." The second principle asserts that "the enjoyment of the highest attainable standard of health is one of the fundamental rights of every human being." And the sixth principle asserts that "healthy development of the child is of basic importance; the ability to live harmoniously in a changing total environment is essential to such development."

This definition obviously has some of the features we would expect in a eudaimonistic conception of health. One is the inclusion of both its negative and positive dimensions: health is declared not to be "merely" the absence of disease or infirmity. Another is the identification of health with *complete* physical, mental, and social well-being. The social dimension of this is reiterated in the sixth principle, in its assertion that "the ability to live harmoniously in a changing total environment" is essential to healthy development in children.

The notion of "complete" health has been the source of a good deal of criticism— including the charge that, if taken seriously in a public-policy sense, it would medicalize every aspect of distributive justice or governmental social programs. Given the prominence of the definition, as well as the fact that some of the criticism of it has come from prominent philosophers working in bioethics (see the overview in Bok, 2008), it is probably wise to say a word here about its relation to the eudaimonistic conception of health I will propose.

Traits versus states. In the first place, notice the World Health Organization's incautious reference to health as a *state* of well-being rather than a stable trait. I will have more to say about trait-health later, but note here only that speaking about a "state" of well-being leads us away from one of the central concerns of eudaimonistic theories—namely, the stable physical, psychological, and behavioral traits or dispositions that are characteristic of organic flourishing as a human being. Without the persistence of underlying healthy traits, the occurrent states themselves are unstable, unreliable, and often damaging. It is the underlying traits of health that allow us to flourish in a dynamic relationship with an unpredictable environment.

In the eudaimonistic conception of health proposed here, trait-health will be distinguished from occurrent health *conditions*, and both will be factors in overall judgments about individual and population health. This is not necessarily inconsistent with the World Health Organization's definition: "state" as it occurs in that text could in principle be understood to include both traits and occurrent conditions. But without that gloss, the connection to a eudaimonistic conception of health is lost.

The ambiguity of "complete" well-being. The second source of trouble lies in the World Health Organization's reference to health as *complete* well-being. On the one hand, the reference might mean only that health is to be defined positively as well as negatively, and that its sources are to be found along physiological and psychological dimensions, heavily influenced by socioeconomic circumstances.

That fits well enough with eudaimonism, and also seems uncontroversial—unless one reads it as an attempt to construct the definition of health in ethical terms rather than in terms of physiological and psychological science.[2] But it is not necessary to read the notion of complete *health* in this way, as the subsequent discussion in this chapter and the next two chapters will show.

As noted earlier, ancient eudaimonistic sources sometimes do run the analogy between health and human flourishing all the way out to the vanishing point of perfection. But as also noted earlier, focusing on this vanishing point has little relevance to theories of basic justice, and that subject seems to have been in the background of ancient eudaimonistic theories. Those philosophers were well aware of the distinction between what we can justifiably require and what we can justifiably admire. Basic justice is about justifiable requirements, and using a eudaimonistic conception of health will not necessarily import a standard of perfect health into normative discussions about basic justice and health.

1.2. *Health as inseparable from basic virtue and well-being*

A eudaimonistic conception of health is closely correlated on its positive side with contemporary psychology—both with respect to psychopathology, where it is easiest to see, and with respect to at least some of the work on happiness and well-being (Keyes, 2009). And in both contemporary psychology and eudaimonism, there is a close connection between healthy human development and basic character traits associated with virtue. Unsurprisingly, a discussion of that connection will overlap substantially with a description of the circumstances of habilitation for basic justice.

Sociality. For example, sociality is a part of health, both in eudaimonistic accounts and in contemporary psychology. This means that we need not quarrel, scientifically, with a eudaimonistic framework in which healthy human development

---

[2] Some of the debate in bioethics about the definition of health has been about whether there is a purely descriptive, value-free, scientific definition of health, or whether health is implicitly a normative concept connected to notions of what is good for humans—and ultimately what is ethically good. Christopher Boorse is a leading advocate of the attempt to give a purely descriptive definition, free of ethical content. And his attempts to do this have generated a good deal of criticism. An overview of this debate, spanning more than twenty years, which gives a good picture of its intensity as well as its content, may be found in Boorse's "A Rebuttal on Health," in J. M. Humber and R. F. Almeder (eds.), *What Is Disease?* (1997, 1–134). It is notable that although Boorse still wants to define health as the absence of pathology, he now includes both a space for "positive health" and an environmental dimension in his definition (at 13.) The definition I will offer here gives a much more expansive role for both of those elements than Boorse does, but it is no less purely descriptive or scientific in nature. After all, it does not follow from the fact that eudaimonistic ethical theory uses a given definition of health that that definition is an ethical one—any more than it would follow that because eudaimonistic ethical theory proceeds in terms of standard definitions of logical validity and soundness that those definitions are ethical ones.

produces the capacity for empathy with and attachments to those closest to us, along with a gradually developed concern for and delight in the well-being of others for their own sakes, and simple norms of fairness, reciprocity, and reliability internalized from sustained social relationships with others. The absence of such developed functional abilities and stable patterns of behavior is understood in eudaimonistic theory to be a health-related deficiency. Their lack is understood as pathological in contemporary psychology. The extreme example is the psychopath.

Agency. Our understanding is similar with respect to the development of agency, when that is understood simply as purposive behavior, with the practical abilities necessary for at least occasional success in achieving important goals, and with the specific form of energy needed for initiating and sustaining effective purposive activity (call it agentic-energy). Such agency, when it is healthy, may begin in infancy with largely egoistic agendas, but they are quickly coordinated with the demands of sociality. The lack of such socialized agency is seen as a health-related deficiency in contemporary psychology as well as in eudaimonistic ethical theory.

Emotion. Simultaneously with the development of agency, healthy human development involves the differentiation and modulation of primal affective responses through self-awareness, awareness of causal connections between external events and internal affective states, and striving for congruence between the norms of sociality and the aims of agency generally. Thus, in healthy adults, as health is understood in both contemporary psychology and eudaimonistic theory (though the jargon used varies from writer to writer), primal affect becomes emotion proper and is more or less successfully yoked to sociality and agency.

Self-awareness, language acquisition, communication, and cooperation. Moreover, the development of a self-concept and the acquisition of language, together with the abilities to communicate, coordinate, and cooperate with others— which are important both to agency and to sociality—develop with considerable momentum in healthy human beings, in the course of ordinary childhood social interactions. Deficiencies in these capabilities, or in their development, are health issues as well for both developmental psychology and eudaimonistic ethical theory.

Strong, stable, homeostatic traits. Habilitation into healthy forms of sociality, agency, emotion, self-awareness, language use, communication, and cooperation proceeds incrementally, and recursively, building upon itself. For that, one needs to achieve forms of health that are immune from or resistant to reversals, and resilient when immunity or resistance fails. One needs traits (persistent dispositions) as opposed to mere states of being or mere behaviors. One needs robustly homeostatic traits—physical, psychological, and social. Without such self-corrective mechanisms, one's health is fragile and subject to reversals that make habilitation difficult or perhaps impossible. Eudaimonistic theories emphasize both physical and psychological strength and stability with respect to sudden reversals and adversity. Psychotherapeutic theories emphasize this as well, through training directed at the development of resilience, defense mechanisms, patterns of adjustment, and cognitive behavior therapy.

A stable, favorable social environment. When one's social environment is constantly and dangerously in flux—in ways that cause reversals—habilitation into health is difficult or impossible to sustain. Ancient eudaimonistic theorists were of course aware of the importance of making health-related traits strong rather than vulnerable. And they were aware of the connection between such strength and social circumstances. They differed among themselves—even perhaps among advocates of the same version of eudaimonistic theory—about the extent to which we could expect healthy character to become fragile and vulnerable in tragic circumstances. The same sort of interest in the topic, and ambivalence about it, can be found in contemporary psychology.

With this much in the background, it should be clear why a eudaimonistic account of health will be plausible if it can answer some further questions about how it might appropriately be limited to matters of basic justice. I turn to those questions now.

2. A Unified Conception of Health, Positive and Negative

As long as we focus on a purely negative conception of health—defined as the absence of disease, disorder, damage to vital functions, interrupted development, and physical or psychological distress—we will leave out many matters that are of the first importance to both science and ethics. Those matters concern the obvious, two-way causal connections between the absence of ill health and the presence of good health—good health defined as various levels of strength, stability, resilience, and so forth. And of course the same thing happens if we focus exclusively on the positive side: the causal connections between the positive and negative sides of the ledger recede into the background.

Strength, stability, and energy. In practice, of course, the presence and importance of such connections are well recognized. The positive and negative sides of health may be discussed separately, but the causal connections between them are acknowledged. The elimination of physical disease, deficit, disorder, or distress is not enough to stabilize and sustain physical health. *Merely* being free of pathology leaves a person highly vulnerable to relapse. To eliminate or reduce such vulnerability, people need the positive physical strengths, resilience, and energy that, in the available environments, make them immune to, or resistant to, relapses into the negative territory of ill health. They need habilitation directed toward acquiring or strengthening such capabilities. And they need rehabilitation not only when things go wrong on the negative side of the ledger, but also when their positive health is damaged in ways that undermine health defined negatively. The same connection is standardly recognized for mental health: eliminating ill health doesn't by itself guarantee the stability of health defined negatively; for stability, positive strengths are required.

Feedback loops and spirals. Further, there is a large body of science that connects physical and psychological health to each other in feedback loops (downward spirals) that run through persistent traits and conditions and/or social circumstances: for example, physical ill health that leads to lowered energy; low energy that leads to lowered initiative and activity; which in turn leads to increasing difficulties with work and/or relationships with family and friends; which in turn leads to inertia, ennui, and depression; which in turn leads to unhealthy patterns of behavior; which increases physical ill health and starts the cycle again. It is clear that unless this cycle is broken by more than simply removing the physical ill health that starts it all, physical health will not be stable. Similar downward spirals begin with mental ill health.

A unified and limited conception. With respect to habilitation, we clearly need an account of human health that recognizes all these causal connections between the negative and positive sides of the ledger for both physical and mental health. This unified conception of health—positive and negative, physical and mental— restricted to areas in which there are such reciprocal causal connections, seems a plausible candidate for the level of health that might be required by basic justice. For other purposes, we can of course project strategies for habilitation all the way out to some ideal form of health and well-being, far beyond what seems plausible to require of ourselves and others. For basic justice, however, a more modest goal is needed, and I will argue in later chapters that restricting our attention to the areas of health in which we can document the causal connections that create downward or upward spirals allows us to set an appropriate goal for basic justice. Optimal progress toward perfect well-being is not the issue here.

This unitary but limited conception of health—one that emphasizes both the causal and conceptual connections between its negative and positive sides, as well as the fact that those connections do not run all the way out to ideal well-being—already exists in major areas of health research and practice.

2.1. *Well-being and the public health tradition*

The concern for positive health of the sort just described has been one of the central elements of research and public policy aimed at explaining, predicting, or improving the health of populations. This shows itself pointedly in work by demographers, economists, sociologists, and medical scientists who investigate the correlations between health negatively defined and a long list of other factors: socioeconomic status, education, work, recreation, environmental factors, occupational hazards, social norms, so-called lifestyle behaviors, and various measures of subjective well-being. Study of these "other" factors often yields recommendations for a better level of positive health—wellness, or fitness, or immunity from environmental hazards.

An appropriate sense of caution about this sort of work on positive health comes from considering its history, which has a very large dark side. Think of attempts to give physiological, genetic, or evolutionary justifications for brutally repressive social policies with respect to sex, race, social status, poverty, and disability. Think about early twentieth-century eugenics, and not only under the Nazis. The public health tradition—whether defined negatively or positively or both—is extremely hazardous, morally, when it is severed from a defensible normative account of basic justice, supported by a defensible comprehensive ethical theory.

So it is important to keep it connected to a normative tradition in ethics, such as eudaimonism, limited by a defensible concept of basic justice. But the point here is that connecting rigorous empirical work in medical and social science to a unitary and limited conception of health, defined both negatively and positively, is nothing new.

2.2. *Well-being and clinical medicine*

The same is true of clinical medicine. There too the causal connections between ill health and good health have long been recognized, both in research and practice. The physiology underlying all areas of medicine supports the standard practice of doing much more than merely eliminating disease, deficit, disability, or distress. Stabilizing people at that (neutral) level, so that they can then be substantially strengthened and stabilized at a higher, positive level of health is an obvious and necessary health care goal. Stable forms of strength, resilience, resistance, and immunity are necessary to prevent relapse. And it is standardly recognized that such levels of positive health need to be high enough to be maintained in a reasonable range of challenging environments. Good medical habilitation and rehabilitation aims at achieving such positive health.

Moreover, there has always been a steady stream of basic science and clinical science aimed at understanding the factors involved in producing good health. That work supports preventive clinical medicine and "wellness" regimens of many sorts, as well as rehabilitation—both physical and psychological.

Wars, epidemics, and widely publicized examples of ill health often bring these sorts of positive health concerns to light in a vivid way. Immunology, for example, gets attention in the context of epidemics of influenza, smallpox, polio, and diseases for which we are still seeking vaccines. Rehabilitation medicine also gets attention in the context of epidemics—and sometimes just in the context of celebrated cases. Polio is an example of both, at least in the United States, which had repeated epidemics in the early twentieth century and a particularly celebrated case in Franklin Delano Roosevelt.

The signature injuries of various wars (shock from physical trauma, amputations, shell shock, traumatic brain injury, post-traumatic stress disorder) get attention during and after the fact in the same two ways involving positive health. One is habilitative, by giving attention to the ways in which such injuries can either be prevented or made survivable—for example, by getting agreements between belligerents not to use chemical or biological warfare; by improving the speed with which traumatic injuries are fully treated; by the use of better body armor. The other is rehabilitative, by giving attention to the ways in which people with survivable injuries of these sorts can be restored.

All of this is tied to achieving a limited level of positive health—the level necessary for restoring and sustaining the physical and psychological stability, strength, resilience, and immunity needed to keep one above the negative side of the health ledger.

What is disappointing about current practice, however, is a lack of clarity and consistency (to put it charitably) about the level of positive health that clinical medicine should pursue—and the level of it that health insurance should support. This lack of clarity and consistency has often meant that systematic work on the positive side of the health ledger has been postponed. Examples of this sort of postponement are easily found in the mental health area. (For perspicuous overviews, see Jahoda, 1958; Vaillant, 2003.)

Furthermore, research and clinical work on even this limited form of positive health seem fragile—often considered along with other "enhancements" that are only indirectly related to genuine health matters. We see this in the way long-term physical rehabilitation is folded into the economic goals of work-related rehabilitation, vocational training, or education. Or the ways in which long-term psychological and behavioral rehabilitation is folded into education, occupational medicine, crime prevention programs, and goals for deinstitutionalization. Or the ways in which immunization programs come to be regarded as optional—a matter of individual risk assessment and choice, along with other lifestyle choices, rather than strictly health-related ones.

The problem is that once matters of positive health are regarded as "enhancements," they often seem to have no predefined common sense or ethical boundaries. Thus we wonder where to draw the line between reconstructive and cosmetic surgery; between legitimate and illegitimate strength training in sports; between ethically objectionable and unobjectionable performance enhancement for various occupations. Psychotherapy on the positive side of the ledger is now frequently distanced from a discussion of health and directed to life-coaching or counseling for wellness, happiness, and life satisfaction.

Moreover, "positive" clinical medicine and psychology have a dark side that rivals the one for public health. Medical quackery and pseudoscience to prevent moral degeneracy in individuals is appalling enough when confined to the treatment of a few isolated individuals. But when such things become popularized as standard treatments, and when such standards bear a suspicious resemblance to independently motivated social norms that underlie racism, sexism, homophobia, or other forms of oppression, programs designed to pursue positive health can do widespread damage. It looks very much as though the worst of this in the history of clinical medicine has been connected to various conceptions of perfect health and virtue, which are then used to identify various forms of "degeneracy" or even disease or deficit that are in need of correction.

All of this tends to reinforce the practice of marginalizing or excluding altogether from clinical medicine much of what eudaimonistic theorists think of as health—leaving it in the hands of people interested in "soft" things like flourishing, a good life, wellness, holistic health, happiness, joy, and quality-of-life issues rather than health, strictly defined. The range of things that health insurance schemes will pay for is a reflection of this—and of the fear that extending the definition of health into the positive side of things will be completely unmanageable.

3. The Science of Mental Health, Happiness, and Virtue

The recent growth of positive psychology illustrates two things of particular interest here. One is the way in which rigorous work on the positive side of the health ledger can stay closely connected to a limited and unified conception of health, defined both positively and negatively, along comprehensive physiological, psychological, and environmental dimensions. This is useful support for the conception of health that I am advancing here with respect to basic justice.

The other thing that positive psychology illustrates is the way in which health can be largely left behind in favor of studying the traits and states historically identified with happiness and virtue *beyond* what we typically think of as health. Here positive psychology illustrates something problematic for present purposes, since it seems to loosen its contact with health science and practice. The leading example of this is probably the focus on happiness as subjective well-being, where that is meant to encompass all aspects of "thinking and feeling positively about one's life" (Diener and Biswas-Diener, 2008). Consider that problematic part first.

3.1. *Positive psychology beyond health and basic justice*

It is obviously unreasonable to think that we could *require* of each other, as a matter of basic justice, that we be optimistic, full of hope, joy, and happiness generally; that we actually flourish at some ideal level—except, possibly, at the level of creating and maintaining capabilities for *pursuing* the ideal. Positive psychology addresses such capabilities by investigating various elements of enduring psychological stability and strength (courage, persistence, resilience, optimism, and so forth) as well as the positive affective states that often supervene upon psychological stability and strength (joy, "flow," subjective happiness, and life satisfaction). Some of this work on stability and strength is obviously connected to matters of basic mental or physical health. But mention of this is oddly deemphasized in surveys of the field. Rather, those surveys suggest that much of positive psychology tracks the traditional interests of philosophical and religious conceptions of the good life—in levels leading up to an ideal one, as opposed to a basically decent one—rather than the traditional interests of the health sciences.

This focus on issues beyond health is apparent in two leading handbooks that give an overview of the field of positive psychology. Consider, for example, the massive *Character Strengths and Virtues: A Handbook and Classification* (Peterson and Seligman, 2004). Written and edited by major contributors to the field, the book is framed by the results of an extensive survey of historical, religious, and philosophical material on virtue and moral character. This is used to develop a theoretical structure and classification scheme for work in positive psychology. The editors' long-range ambition is to develop an equivalent, on the positive side, to the American Psychiatric Association's widely used and regularly updated reference work on mental illness and psychopathology. That would lead one to believe that the book's target is mental *health* rather than mental illness. But in the index to the book's more than 800 pages, there is no reference to the term "health" at all, mental or physical, and only a single, one-page reference to psychopathology.

Of course, in one sense this is perfectly appropriate. After all, scientific psychology can perfectly well investigate mental phenomena other than positive health. In particular, it can investigate various aspects of happiness as that term is understood in various cultural contexts, as well as various traits of character, and their strength levels, generally identified as intellectual or moral virtues. There is no particular reason, a priori, why a classification scheme for positive psychology must be tethered to a conception of health rather than well-being generally. Moreover, there is no particular reason, a priori, to think that positive psychology should examine normative theories of justice and ethics for anything more than leads on what topics to pursue, and how to classify its results.

The subordination of health found in the organizational scheme of *Character Strengths and Virtues* is thus not implausible. The book groups traits under six major headings, each corresponding to a constellation of items identified, cross-culturally, as a core virtue. These core virtues are defined in terms of various kinds of strength— for example, wisdom, courage, temperance, justice, and so forth (Peterson and Seligman, 2004, 29–30). The book's proposed research agenda for positive psychology is nominally fitted to those virtues but proceeds directly to the study of the strength and weakness of character traits under each heading, their affective dimensions, and the situational factors that influence both traits and associated affect.

It is probably understood by the authors, as so obvious that it needs no comment, that all of this taken together will *include* mental health. It will thus include the aspects of it (if any) that are relevant to normative theories of basic justice at issue here. But what cannot be missed is that it also includes much more than health. Moreover, it is not helpful, in any obvious way, in sorting out the material relevant to our purposes from the material that is not relevant. (Something similar is true for the research agenda for eudaimonistic ethical theory: clearly it includes much more than the material relevant for basic justice, but not immediately clear is which parts are relevant. Theories of basic justice still have to construct accounts of basic goods, and basic health.)

A roughly similar choice of topics in positive psychology shows up in the current edition of the *Oxford Handbook of Positive Psychology* (Snyder and Lopez, 2009). This handbook is also large, with sixty-two chapters in its 600-plus pages. Eight of these chapters address matters of mental health directly, and some of them do so in a way that connects to the limited, unified conception of eudaimonistic health proposed here. But of the remaining fifty-four chapters, almost all fit naturally into the framework described in *Character Strengths and Virtues*: their connection to mental health is implicit, and implicitly for a very wide agenda for it which (like eudaimonism itself) stretches from matters of concern to basic justice out to forms of flourishing that are clearly beyond anything we could plausibly require of ourselves and others.

3.2. *Positive psychology for mental health and well-being*

Positive psychology does, however, include a complex, so far largely programmatic, stream of work from many investigators that is directly relevant to a eudaimonistic conception of complete health[3]—in which the causal connections and

---

[3] A term borrowed from the World Health Organization's definition of health; it means here simply a unified account of health, including physiological, psychological, and social factors, along negative and positive dimensions, ranging over health-states from worst possible to best possible. Used this way, it coincides with the conception of the health scale developed in Chapters 4 and 5.

correlations between mental and physical, positive and negative dimensions of health are systematically explored. In the *Oxford Handbook of Positive Psychology* cited earlier, a good deal of this work is referenced by Corey L. M. Keyes, in the chapter called "Toward a Science of Mental Health" (Keyes, 2009, 89–96). Keyes summarizes the research (some of it his own) on "mental health conceived of as a constellation of dimensions of subjective well-being, specifically hedonic-eudaemonic measures of subjective well-being." He defines a mental health continuum ranging from languishing, through moderate mental health, to flourishing. Languishing is defined as the zero point at which diagnosable mental illness is absent, but one remains "stuck, stagnant, or empty, devoid of [much] positive functioning."

Keyes's own work then focuses on getting subjects' self-reported assessments of their well-being on both hedonic (affective) and eudaimonistic (capability and functioning) scales, operationalizing the definitions of languishing, moderate, and flourishing levels with a combination of the two scales. "Flourishing" individuals exhibit high levels on at least one of the two measures of hedonic well-being, and high levels on at least six of the eleven measures of positive functioning (eudaimonistic well-being). Languishing individuals exhibit low levels on at least one measure of hedonic well-being and low levels on at least six of the eleven measures of positive functioning. Adults who meet neither the criteria for flourishing or languishing are scored as "moderately mentally healthy" (90). He goes on to report evidence that flourishing is the appropriate target level for mental health because, at that level, there is a strong correlation between mental health and physiological health (92). And of course, directly from the eleven measures of positive functioning themselves, there is a strong correlation between mental health and functioning in work environments, personal relationships, and so forth.

Keyes makes a plausible case for the usefulness, and limitations, of such self-reported assessments as indicators of more objective determinations of individual well-being along these two dimensions. This is a point of considerable interest for public policy, since it must often work with self-reported data. (A good deal of the public health information collected by governments comes from self-reports. An example is the National Health Information Survey conducted annually in the United States by the National Center for Health Statistics, part of the Centers for Disease Control.)

Other work to which Keyes refers, and other chapters in the *Oxford Handbook*, are also of interest for present purposes.

Eudaimonistic well-being. For one thing, there is currently some conflict in positive psychology about whether to pursue the study of subjectively estimated eudaimonistic well-being (defined and assessed in terms of capabilities and functioning that may or may not be directly correlated to positive affect) in addition to the study of subjectively estimated positive affective states indicative of happiness. It appears that this dispute is not about the importance of both of these dimensions of well-being itself. Rather, it is about whether the large body of literature on hedonic measures should now be revised to include both eudaimonistic and hedonic ones.

It seems clear enough in principle that scientific psychology should do both, with any well-validated measurement devices available, including but not limited to subjective self-reports. The argument for including functional well-being is obvious: mental *health* is mostly about positive functioning and appropriate or functional affect, just as mental illness is mostly about dysfunctional behavior and inappropriate or dysfunctional affect. And it is fair to say that conceptually, health generally, physical or mental, is ultimately defined in terms of functional abilities and well-being rather than in terms of subjective happiness or unhappiness. That does not mean that the subjective dimension is unimportant. It simply means that if positive psychology is going to concern itself with mental health at all, it needs to concern itself with eudaimonistic well-being.

Inevitably, then, the mental health agenda within positive psychology will be aligned loosely with the eudaimonistic tradition in naturalistic ethics. This does not commit psychology to adopting a specific normative agenda in ethics. It simply acknowledges the greater usefulness of some rather than other philosophical ancestors.

It seems a natural step to go from this to giving more emphasis to the health-oriented agenda of positive psychology and connecting it explicitly to a conception of complete health—that is, an integrated conception of physiological and psychological factors, along negative and positive dimensions with respect to health, together with the environmental factors that make it possible. And in fact, work along these lines is going on. Some of it is summarized by Keyes in the article just cited. But there is a good deal more, some of it on the point of reciprocal causal connections between physical and psychological health (Snyder and Lopez, 2009, section 8, "Biological Approaches").

All of this is promising, though it is very far from a tidy, thoroughly unified conception of complete health. And for purposes of basic justice, we are not yet much closer to an understanding of the point at which declines in health must become a matter of concern for normative theories of basic justice, and at which further improvements in health can reasonably be assigned to something other than basic justice.

4. Health, Happiness, and Basic Justice

The existing philosophical literature on the nature of happiness or a good life is replete with discussions that mention health in passing. Unfortunately, like the literature on the same subject in positive psychology, it gives very little guidance on the specific questions we need answered for this project: namely, what sorts of health-related habilitation can be regarded as matters of basic justice for individuals, and what sorts contribute most importantly to creating and sustaining the individual behavior and social institutions necessary for a basically just society.

4.1. *Health and moral development*

The basic equipment for a moral life. As previously noted, it is clear enough that a eudaimonistic conception of health tracks a scientific conception of moral development that is (at a very basic level) common to plausible normative theories generally; it is not simply eudaimonism that recommends basic prosocial, cooperative, and productive traits and behaviors. Observational and experimental science gives all those normative theories a reason for supporting health in at least those respects, as a matter of basic justice. Habilitation into basic health, covering both its physical and psychological factors, negatively and positively defined, will inevitably include habilitation for basic moral development.

But it is not so clear where, if at all, we should draw the line and say that progress toward better and better health will *cease* to track moral development in this way. As noted earlier, this is not even agreed-upon within eudaimonistic theory itself, let alone normative theory generally. So we still need a theory-independent way of indicating (say, for dental care) what level of health is of basic importance for virtue, or moral life, or the social structures that support it, and thus for basic justice.

The basic equipment for a good life. Similarly, we do not yet have a way of deciding what level of health is necessary for things that lie beyond a life of morally good behavior—specifically, a good life, a life worth living, a fulfilling or happy life. Conceptions of the good life vary a good deal more than conceptions of basic moral development. Is the basic habilitative task for all of them related to health in some way? Can we specify a basic level of health that will be the necessary basis for the full range of capabilities that might be required by any (normatively defensible) given conception of a good life? If not, then the conception of eudaimonistic health will not be sufficient for present meta-theoretical purposes.

4.2. *Health, well-being, and lives that go well*

Well-being. I am reasonably confident that the conception of health being developed in this book is consistent with accounts of human happiness and a good life meant to answer the question(s) "What does it mean to say that the life you have led, or are leading, is a happy one, a fortunate one, a flourishing one, a good one?"[4]

---

[4] Daniel M. Haybron, *The Pursuit of Unhappiness* (2008, 29–32), distinguishes that question from "What does it means to *be* happy, in a purely psychological sense?" I will deal with the psychological or

The major candidates for an answer (once they are adjusted to accommodate important objections) are essentially theories of well-being, connected closely to ancestral versions of eudaimonistic ethical theory. That connection will guarantee that the habilitation framework, with its emphasis on health and healthy agency, is sufficient for well-being *with respect to basic justice*—though not sufficient with respect to an ideal of *perfect* well-being. Consider these general possibilities:

Hedonistic theories, in which well-being consists in a favorable balance of pleasant over unpleasant experience, whether such experience has its source in the individual's desires, preferences, and choices, or not. Obvious objections to be met include cases in which such experience is not authentic (e.g., because it is a psychosomatic fantasy provided by an "Experience Machine"); is self-defeating or otherwise perverse; is not congruent with fully informed desires or preferences or choices; is not congruent with basic justice, and so forth.

Desire- or preference-satisfaction theories, in which well-being consists in a favorable balance of fulfillment over unfulfillment of the individual's desires, whether such fulfillment is, or is even meant to be, directly pleasurable or not. Obvious objections to be met, again, include cases in which the desires might be inauthentic, self-defeating, not fully informed, not equivalent to rational need-satisfaction, or not congruent with basic justice.

Life-satisfaction accounts, in which well-being comes from an affirmative response to one's life as a whole, past and present, whether or not it has been especially pleasant, or especially full of desire-fulfillment. Such satisfaction may range from an affectless absence of regret to intensely positive satisfaction with the way one's life has gone, overall. Obvious objections to be met include cases in which such global judgments might not be autonomous (but rather, for example, are produced by psychological or social factors of which one is unaware), or not fully informed about the range of possibilities that were actually available, or not corrected for biases and other deficiencies in deliberation and choice, and so forth.

Potential-realization accounts, in which well-being consists in the realization of one's particular possibilities, or one's generic possibilities as a human being. This includes, but is not limited to, the sort of teleological naturalism found in ancient Greek eudaimonism. Obvious objections to be met include cases in which the realization of one's potential occurs in a life full of misery (pain, frustration, or regret), or can be congruent with ignorance, lack of autonomy, or great evil.

List theories, in which well-being consists in meeting threshold levels of a disparate set of goods. Obvious objections to be met here include charges that the list is ad hoc, that the thresholds are arbitrary, and that some sort of unitary account will be needed in any case to resolve such charges.

---

affective sense of happiness in the section following this one. The way of setting up these issues and laying out the overview of alternatives roughly follows the one given in Haybron's book, on pp. 29–36, though the details of my exposition are distinct from his.

On my reading of the philosophical literature on these matters, when advocates for one or another of these general accounts work out a plausible conception of a good life that meets the obvious objections, those conceptions wind up endorsing something that is consistent with the general form of eudaimonistic health proposed here for the habilitation framework. The differences lie in matters of emphasis and in the fact that an account of a good life will usually be extended beyond the concerns of basic justice.

It is therefore not hard to see how the habilitative requirements for well-being under each of these headings would be on the same axis as those of eudaimonistic health—though perhaps at different points along that axis. But it seems evident that anyone habilitated to a substantial level of physical and psychological positive health will thereby have the *capacity* (in some circumstances) for a favorable balance of pleasant over unpleasant experience, the fulfillment of a satisfactory level of fully informed desires, a fully informed, autonomous and positive form of life-satisfaction, some basic level of the realization of one's potential, and threshold levels of at least some items on any plausible list of elements of a good life. It should therefore not be hard, in principle, to define a level of habilitation into health that adequately represents what is required for a basic level of well-being (and thus basic justice) that includes all of these accounts.

4.3. *Health and happiness*

One thing that remains so far unaddressed is an important question about happiness as a purely psychological, affective state.[5] Philosophical accounts of well-being other than hedonism tend to deemphasize the intrinsic good of sensory pleasures and pains, somatic-affective "feelings," passions, emotions, and moods. Instead, philosophers generally choose to emphasize the instrumental role those things can play in well-being and happiness, and even that instrumental role is usually presented as dependent on the associated cognitive and intentional content of emotional states rather than their purely affective qualities. (The so-called cognitive theory of emotion has ancient roots.)

This deemphasis persists even though everyone acknowledges that positive affect itself, not just the cognitive and intentional content associated with it, is fundamental to ordinary conceptions of well-being, happiness, and a good life, just as its opposites on the negative side—pain, suffering, bad feelings, negative

---

[5] The discussion throughout this section is indebted to Daniel Haybron's discussion of some of these issues in *The Pursuit of Unhappiness* (2008), though his concern is not with the line of argument being developed here.

emotions, bad moods—are fundamental to ordinary conceptions of *un*happiness, and an *un*satisfactory life.

The soft-pedaling of the purely affective dimension of happiness comes in part from the pressure philosophers are under to respond to several important types of objections to incautious accounts of affective well-being:

a. the objection that strong affective experience on either side of the ledger frequently distorts sound perception, deliberation, judgment, and decision making;

b. the objection that decision making with a strong affective component can overwhelm virtuous intentions and virtuous traits of character, leading to behavior that is irrational, or inconsistent with justice;

c. the objection that ordinary conceptions of happiness must be corrected to make clear that genuine well-being and happiness require that justice and the moral virtues generally take priority over pleasant affective states; and

d. the objection that many types of mild-to-moderate affect are essentially trivial matters in any case—things that are of no very great consequence, overall, for how well our lives are going.

The typical result is then that philosophical conceptions of happiness (even hedonistic ones) designed to answer those objections exclude strong and destabilizing affect; trivialize mild, transient affect; and endorse an inventory of well-modulated, stable, and controlled affective states (of both negative and positive sorts) that are compatible with psychological equilibrium and are subordinate to practical wisdom, courage, justice, temperance, and the other moral virtues.

By definition, such calmed-down conceptions of happiness do not attract enthusiasts. That hasn't usually been thought, by philosophers, to be a defect in those conceptions, but rather just another instance of the conflict between poets and philosophers, romantics and rationalists, folk psychology and philosophical psychology. But the ordinary conception of happiness, with its insistence on a strong "feel-good" dimension, will not go away. And it is interesting, in this connection, that for many decades, behavioral science has been undermining some of the assumptions involved in preemptory rejection of the feel-good conception.

In particular, there is now a large body of evidence that even mild and transient affective states are far from trivial and can have strikingly important behavioral consequences—for example, through framing, priming, and biasing effects.[6] There

---

[6] Brian Barry and Russell Hardin (eds.), *Rational Man and Irrational Society* (1982); Daniel Kahneman, *Judgment under Uncertainty* (2001), and *Thinking, Fast and Slow* (2011); John Doris, *Lack of Character* (2002); Dan Ariely, *Predictably Irrational* (2008); Richard H. Thaler and Cass Sunstein, *Nudge* (2008).

is also a developing body of hard evidence that the absence of various affective states has even more striking consequences—for example, by rendering people unable to make decisions at all.[7] And it has given us very good evidence of the connection between the presence of positive affective states and healthy human development throughout the life span.[8]

So it seems clear that the habilitation framework offered in this book, along with its conception of eudaimonistic health, will need to be able to address questions of happiness in this ordinary sense—one that emphasizes its affective dimension. It is important for both behavior and health, so it is important for this meta-theoretical framework to cover the ways in which a normative theory of basic justice might want to address emotional well-being and happiness seriously.

Psychic affirmation and psychic flourishing. Haybron, in *The Pursuit of Unhappiness,* provides an illuminating philosophical analysis of a "purely psychological" account of happiness, meant to be faithful to its ordinary sense in which our emotional and affective states generally are given prominence. He calls his account *the emotional state theory* of happiness and is careful to describe it so as to avoid attempts to reduce it to one or another of the standard accounts of well-being, and at the same time to avoid a list of objections similar to the ones those accounts of affective well-being face. The result is an account of what Haybron calls "psychic affirmation"—a complex psychological state that is not characterized by any particular mood, emotion, feeling, or sensation at all, but rather by the overall predominance, in one's experience, of *positive* "emotional conditions" that are *central* affective states (rather than peripheral or superficial ones), supported by a *disposition* to experience such positive emotional conditions.

Positive emotional states (moods and emotions, mostly) are defined by giving examples drawn from ordinary usage and from positive psychology: "joyfulness, high-spiritedness, peace of mind, etc. . . . rather than their negative counterparts [of] depression, anxiety, fear, feelings of discontent, etc." (Haybron, 2008, 66). *Central* affective states are described this way:

What primarily distinguishes central from peripheral states [either negative or positive ones] is that they *dispose* agents to experience certain [additional] affects rather than others. This, indeed, appears to be their essential characteristic. . . . [But we] can identify at least four other hallmarks of central affective states. First, they are *productive*: they have many and varied causal consequences—generating other affective states, initiating various ideological changes, biasing cognition and behavior, etc. Second, such states tend to be

---

[7] Antonio Damasio, *The Feeling of What Happens* (1999).

[8] The psychiatrist George Vaillant, long-time director of the seven-decade-old Harvard Study of Adult Development, surveys this evidence with respect to spirituality, faith, love, hope, joy, forgiveness, and compassion in his book *Spiritual Evolution* (2008).

persistent: when they occur, they generally last a while. There is a certain inertia to central affective states that peripheral affects seem to lack: they don't vanish without trace the instant the triggering event is over. Third, the relevant states are often *pervasive*: they are frequently confused and nonspecific in character, tending to permeate the whole consciousness, and setting the tone thereof. They are often said to color our experience of life. Finally, they tend to be *profound*: they are somehow deep, including phenomenally, and often visceral in feel. . . . They seem to run all the way through us, in some sense, feeling like states *of* us rather than impingements from without. (130–31)

The *mood propensities* relevant to happiness are forms of emotional resilience (or what I will later call homeostatic resilience): they dispose us to experience positive, rather than negative, central affective states (133–38).

These mood propensities do not immunize us from negative affective experience, but rather tend to bring us back to the positive kind. This is crucial because central affective states, negative and positive, are persistent and perhaps even quasi-dispositional also: they tend to perpetuate or even exaggerate themselves or related states. So the presence of positive mood propensities (and their preponderance over any such negative propensities?), will be necessary for sustaining the preponderance of the positive central affective experience that is definitive of happiness on the emotional state account.

Haybron goes on to group various sorts of positive emotional experience under three categories, in what he conjectures is a descending order of importance for psychic happiness: *attunement* (e.g., peace of mind rather than anxiety, confidence rather than insecurity, and an expansive psychological state rather than a compressed one); *engagement* (e.g., exuberance or vitality rather than listlessness; flow rather than boredom or ennui); and *endorsement* (e.g., joy rather than sadness, cheerfulness rather than irritability). He contends that it is hopeless to try to specify a precise ratio of positive to negative experience along these dimensions that yields a precise boundary between happiness and unhappiness. Rather, he is content with a vague threshold:

To be happy, then, is for one's emotional condition to be broadly positive—involving stances of attunement, engagement, and endorsement—with negative central affective states and mood propensities only to a minor extent. (147)

That much is what he calls "psychic affirmation." Beyond that lies psychic flourishing rather than simply psychic affirmation (147–48).

This emotional state theory offers an important corrective to those accounts of well-being which more or less ignore the affective dimension of happiness. As Haybron remarks, "Happiness is a matter of central importance for a good life, and an important object of practical concern. To dismiss happiness as a lightweight matter of little import is most likely to be working with a lightweight conception of happiness" (123). His conception of it is certainly not lightweight. It needs to be included in the habilitation framework and its conception of health. (The same would be true of competing philosophical analyses of purely psychological happiness.)

In this case, we can be sure of its inclusion. After all, its connections to standard accounts, particularly eudaimonistic ones, are clear: the important emotional states are not only positive, but central rather than peripheral or superficial; those states are combined with mood propensities, all of which function together as positive psychological traits with considerable strength, stability, and resilience; and a preponderance of such strong, stable, and resilient positive traits is (plausibly) causally connected to sustaining both mental and physical health. All of this should be a leading concern of a eudaimonistic conception of health, and thus of basic justice.

To clinch the connection to eudaimonism, Haybron makes clear that there is one other important similarity. He says, though perhaps with a hint of irritation,

> We should grant that [emotional state] happiness is not as important as some people think it is, and that it ranks firmly beneath virtue in a good life: to sacrifice the demands of good character in the name of personal happiness—or, I would add, personal welfare—can never be justified. We must, above all, act decently, if not well. Or so, at any rate, I am prepared to grant. None of this is incompatible in the least with the aims of this book. (123)

With this, we are firmly back in standard territory.

Once again, however, we lack a clear criterion for deciding what level of well-being, happiness, or a good life can plausibly be regarded as a matter of basic justice. But once again, it appears that the key to getting that criterion lies in getting a unified conception of health—positive and negative, physiological and psychological.

The reasoning is simple: (1) It is wholly implausible to think that *ill* health is not part of the subject of basic justice. (2) So if it turns out that some elements of *good* health (call them physical and psychological strengths) are necessary for removing or sustaining the absence of illness, those factors of good health will also be part of the subject matter of basic justice. (3) We have good reason to think that various elements of psychological well-being are necessary for sustaining physical and psychological strengths—and thus necessary for preventing declines toward ill health. (4) Such strengths are thereby part of the subject a matter of basic justice. (5) And if the same thing is true about purely psychological happiness (psychic affirmation or psychic flourishing), it too will be part of the subject matter of basic justice.

Inclusion in the subject matter covered by the habilitation framework does not mean, of course, that competing normative theories of justice will have to agree on all the details of treating complete health as a matter of basic justice. But it does mean that all normative theories will have to confront the issue of *how much* should be provided, *to* whom, and *by* whom.

4

Good Health as Reliably Competent Functioning

The eudaimonistic account of human health sketched in the previous chapter suggests that healthy human development itself will supply an important range of the motivational traits required by basic justice, though perhaps no more than that. This is so for the following conjunction of reasons.

First, there is a limited conception of health (basic health) within the eudaimonistic conception of "complete" health. That internal partition comes at the point at which further improvements in health—in physical and psychological functioning—cease to be significant causal factors in preventing declines toward ill health. (An example of this is the difference between being physically fit in a basic sense and being a world-class decathlete. One can remain fit in that basic sense, and reliably so, without ever having to move toward some version of world-class fitness or virtuosity.) The existence of this limited conception of health offers the possibility that it might match up with a comparably limited conception of justice—that is, basic justice.

Second, nonpathological human development as we understand it, historically and cross-culturally, includes clusters of motivational traits that are of interest to any account of basic justice—dispositions toward mutual restraint, mutual aid, reciprocity, and sociality, for example. This aspect of nonpathological development holds out the possibility that the motivational structure of basically healthy human personality closely matches the motivational structure represented by the norms of basic justice. This parallel is often implicitly noted in developmental psychology and psychiatry in discussions of the mature or integrated personality.

The task of this chapter and the chapters in Part Three will be to assemble the reasons for thinking that basic health in a human being includes stable and strong behavioral traits that are in effect dispositions to follow the most fundamental norms of justice, *as* norms of justice. That is not to say that such dispositions arise quickly or easily. Like health itself, they require a favorable set of physical and psychological endowments in the individual, and a favorable habilitative environment, both physically and socially. Like health itself, they require significant self-habilitative efforts from the individuals themselves. And under certain catastrophic conditions, the acquisition of such fundamental dispositions of justice can be blocked entirely, or entirely transformed into dispositions of *in*justice. Nonetheless, there are convincing reasons for thinking that such dispositions do emerge with considerable momentum in the species-typical course of human development—with the same kind of momentum that characterizes a human being's acquisition of a self-concept, spoken language, or hand-eye coordination—and with only the sort of habilitation necessary for basic health.

An important cautionary note: as far as I can tell, developmental psychologists and psychiatrists do not have a generally agreed upon theory of motivation—in the sense of an explanatory theory, or developmental stage theory, or a psychodynamic theory that comes close to explaining motivation generally. There are theoretical proposals, each of which makes particularly good sense (or in some cases, bad sense) in a particular region of human behavior: language acquisition, motivation attributable to biological evolution, stages of early childhood cognitive development, stages of moral development, hierarchies of survival needs, personality development through childhood and adolescence, and so forth. But attempts to get a covering, foundational, explanatory theory of some sort have so far failed to gain anything like consensus, and some of them, such as those emerging from neuroscience, are so far very sketchy.

This is in sharp contrast to the consensus one finds in purely descriptive, functional accounts of basic good health (physical and psychological) found in developmental psychology and psychiatry. And as I read the literature, there is consensus also about the range of factors that can defeat the development of such basic good health, or destroy or threaten its continuance. This descriptive consensus is sufficient for the argument that follows in this chapter and in Part Three of the book, and it is a happy coincidence that this consensus overlaps almost entirely with descriptive accounts drawn from history, literature, and common wisdom.

This chapter argues that basic good health may be understood as physiological and psychological functioning that is reliably "competent" in a given range of physical and social environments. A central part of such competence has to do with agency, and the individual's coping abilities within those environments. Part Three of the book will argue that the reliably competent functioning found in good health includes behavioral dispositions about the subject matter of basic justice, and that those dispositions *about* basic justice are dispositions *of* basic justice— meaning that those behavioral dispositions reflect the way in which the norms of basic justice are already incorporated into the motivational structure found in basically healthy human agency.

1. Basic Health: An Integrated, Limited General Concept

The argument begins by making clear how the general concept of basic health may be explicated in terms of empirically describable physiological and psychological functioning in a given range of environments. This necessarily includes a focus on the development of the coping abilities characteristic of various forms of agency. And when the subject is basic *good* health, the focus will be on traits that are stable enough, and strong enough, to constitute *reliably competent* coping abilities. Reliable competence is in this case both a minimum and a maximum: anything less than competence is not good health; anything more than merely reliable competence is more than basic good health.

1.1. *Ill health and basic good health*

It is best to start with the negative side of things, since the absence of pathology is the most familiar part of the definition and the most thoroughly worked over in both the clinical and philosophical literature. For present purposes we will say,

Ill health is the presence of functionally significant physical or psychological disease, deficit, disorder, injury, or distress in a given range of environments.

Thus, restoring health *in the illness region* of the health-spectrum is defined negatively—as achieving the *absence* of the elements of ill health.

The conceptual problems with this sort of definition are familiar, and we cope with them well enough for practical purposes. A good deal of attention has been devoted to defining disease and related concepts, for example, in ways which are not moralized or improperly medicalized (as they have historically sometimes been), and which are not infinitely expandable to include increasingly trivial conditions.

For practical purposes, the resolution of these difficulties takes a familiar path. The first step is to describe the clinical manifestations of the presenting condition fully enough to locate them *provisionally* in physiological, psychological, or environmental sources, or in some combination such sources. The next step is to subject that provisional judgment to critical scrutiny so as to avoid inappropriate moralization or medicalization of conditions not directly related to ill health, and to avoid the trivialization of the notion of ill health. With respect to some conditions, this will be a lengthy, iterative process characterized by frequent, all too human errors. But that is a familiar story in all difficult human endeavors.

Basic good health. In the present context, an apt approach to the general concept of *good* health is to ask what (if anything) ill health takes away, or displaces, on the positive (good health) side of the ledger. This focuses attention on the reciprocal causal connections involved—those in which elements of positive or good health are necessary for, or important for, preventing or improving ill health. When a general concept of good health is given in terms of such reciprocal connections, it will necessarily be part of a general concept of basic health in the sense defined here—namely, an integrated concept of health limited (on its upper end) to those positive factors that create or sustain the absence of disease, deficit, disorder, or distress.

So what does ill health take away from good health? Sometimes life itself; sometimes longevity; sometimes the ability to thrive, or to care about thriving; sometimes the ability to be active or effective, or to care about being active and effective; sometimes the ability to flourish or be happy. And it is important to recognize that these things can happen even at the zero point between ill health and positively good health. One can languish at that point, and fail to thrive. Failure to thrive tends to devolve into ill health.

In general terms, survival, longevity, and thriving are at risk whenever physical or psychological functioning in a given environment is significantly unstable or unreliable, vulnerable to damage, underfunded with energy at self-defeating levels, or self-defeating in terms of the direction or process of development or activity. To put it more pointedly, it turns out that anything necessary for physical and psychological thriving is at least indirectly connected to ill health and survival, through a chain of consequences leading to the weakening or destabilization of vital functions. This yields something like the following general concept of basic good health:

Basic good health is the presence, in a given environment, of functionally significant levels of stability and strength in vital functions, together with resistance, immunity, resilience, and regenerative powers with respect to ill health, developmental momentum away from ill health in the generative and regenerative processes characteristic of the human life cycle, and in the energy and activity characteristic of competent functioning humans of a given age, in a given environment.

This may seem almost comically imprecise—and too general to be of practical use. Not to mention that when added to the definition of ill health, it is not only imprecise but lengthy.

I will argue in Chapter 5, however, that these two parts of the general concept of health (ill health and basically good health) give us enough detail to work out a health scale that has two properties of particular interest to normative theories of basic justice: it can solve the indexing problem with respect to health; and it is comprehensive enough to function as the representative good in such theories.

1.2. *Functional significance in a given environment*

For expository purposes here, however, it may be useful to introduce a line of reasoning about what counts as a "functionally significant" physical or psychological condition. On the negative or pathological side of things, the term is obviously meant to capture empirically measurable, un-moralized, nontrivial conditions. But even so, it is a very general term. This can be a challenge for health research and practice, as well as public policy, which need clear, detailed, operationalized, empirical definitions rather than merely gestures toward such definitions.

Modern medicine does have such operationalized definitions in abundance, for various functionally significant illnesses, and uses them successfully for purposes of diagnosis, treatment, insurance reimbursement, and reports to public health departments. And such operationalized definitions on the pathological side of things will "cover" operational needs in the region of *basic* good health as well, by implication from the reciprocal causal connections between the two. If we can agree on diagnostic and treatment manuals for ill health, and we can agree on functionally significant forms of ill health for various environments, then it will follow that those forms of good health that are causally linked to ill health are perforce functionally significant.

With general definitions like this, there are always problems along the margins that escape prompt settlement, especially when there is persistent disagreement among health professionals, or between them and the general public. Such disagreement can be annoying. (The dermatologist says "That's not a disease, you know. That's just a weed in the garden of life.")

Annoyances aside, the way to settle such disagreement is surely to appeal to the objectively definable consequences to the individual (if any), in a given environment, of the sort of functioning involved. We speak of this informally by asking what a given situation actually "calls for," or requires, as opposed to what might be on offer, or desired by the individuals involved. I will return to this issue in Sections 2.1 and 2.2 later in the chapter, in terms of the notions of coping abilities and reliably competent functioning in a given environment. But for the moment it should be clear enough, for example, that what counts as a significant dermatological condition for a screen actor may not be significant for a movie studio accountant, unless the accountant's psychological health is tied up with having clear skin. Conditions that have no direct consequences in terms of physical functioning may nonetheless have direct psychological consequences (anxiety, depression), or direct social consequences (loss of a job), which then may eventually have indirect physical consequences as well.

Similarly, we have to decide what counts as a relevant environment for purposes of assessing functioning. Some people can survive better than others in extreme environments such as the South Pole, or zero gravity. Does that mean that they are just extremely healthy? Or does it mean that the rest of us are unhealthy? Moreover, some people are much fussier than others about apparently minor health conditions—such as discolored teeth or occasional discomfort in a wrist or elbow. Does that mean they are just obsessive about their health? Or that the rest of us are too careless of it?

In sorting out the answers to such questions, we again may properly appeal to the *particular* economic, social, and psychological demands upon *particular* people in the environments in which they must operate. Mood-altering drugs, performance-enhancing drugs, and purely cosmetic surgery sometimes address a functionally significant deficit, injury, or distress; sometimes they address only an insignificant whim; and sometimes they create or reinforce physical or psychological ill health. Paying attention to the particulars helps decide such cases. Performance-enhancing drugs prescribed to pilots in combat are one thing; the same drugs prescribed for college students trying to stay awake to study, after a weekend of partying, are another.

Borderline problems are inevitable when there are borders to begin with. But if the borders are drawn carefully, most cases will fall clearly inside them. The discussion throughout the remainder of the book will often return to the borderline problems, of course. But first it is important to say something more about agency—about healthy agency as it might appear within this general concept of basically good health.

2. Habilitation, Coping Abilities, and Agency

The details of the need for habilitation vary from person to person, if for no other reason than that human beings have diverse sets of physiological and neuropsychological endowments, situated in diverse social and physical environments. However, it is possible to frame a general discussion of one important aspect of the need for habilitation in terms of *coping abilities*. That is so because no matter what our endowments or situations, our most fundamental need is to be able to cope with the world in which we are situated—that is, to survive and thrive in it. That defines both the beginning of our need for habilitative efforts from others and a necessary basic goal for habilitative efforts of our own and others throughout our lives: equipping ourselves and others with the ability to cope with the environment in which we find ourselves, and the environments in which we are likely to find ourselves.

It is plausible to think that human beings who lack agency altogether will also, by that fact alone, lack the ability to cope—at least within the social world humans define for themselves. So the development of agency is a central part of the goal of habilitation, even though it cannot always be accomplished, and even though agency of a single type is not possible across the entire population of human individuals.

2.1. *The range of agency powers in human beings*

Agency, in the sense used here, is much broader than the moral agency discussed in ethics. No human being is a moral agent at birth, although almost all are agents in some sense. The functional abilities of moral agency develop slowly, if at all, through habilitation under favorable circumstances. Some human beings never achieve it. Questions of distributive justice, however, arise with regard to all of us, and to other beings like us. Normative theories that begin by posing questions about how "persons" interact, and then slide easily into identifying persons with moral agents, are likely to push other human agents permanently to the edges of the theory. The result will be an account of basic justice that is unsatisfying to people whose focus is on human beings generally, or perhaps all sentient beings. Framing questions in terms of habilitation will avoid some of these problems if one is careful to think about the varieties of agency found in the world.[1]

Impersonal animal agency. For example, like many other animals, some human beings lack self-awareness and have only limited apprehension of the past, or of future possibilities. Nonetheless, they may still be able to develop an impressive form of agency in the sense of relentless purposive behavior. They may not be well suited for thriving within an elaborately developed human social world. And, unlike many animals who have a very brief developmental phase, human beings with this sort of impersonal animal agency will not even be able to thrive in societies of similar agents, human or nonhuman, without an elaborately reconstructed social world. This will present wrenching problems of justice to the extent that the human social world is unwilling or unable to accommodate this form of agency in ways that sustain it, rather than extinguish it.

Personal animal agency. The situation will be somewhat less stark for those human beings who, like many other animals, become aware of themselves as distinct from their environments, who become aware of the possibility that some of their goal-directed activity can be self-directed, but who do not become language users and thus have to operate exclusively with the forms of memory, imagination, and communication possible without language. Even so, such human beings may achieve a rudimentary form of reflective agency and autonomy as well as significant personalities and social abilities.

They lack significant powers that we associate with rational and moral agency, however. They lack the ability to organize their experience and represent it to themselves as a personal history that can be explained; they lack the ability to represent their trial and error learning to themselves in terms of rules or general relationships between things; and they lack the ability to organize their goal-directed activity and to represent it to themselves in terms of a coherent plan for the future.

---

[1] For an elegant and compact summary of her account of the general faculty of human reason, or agency, and its relation to both rational principles and reasons for action, see Christine M. Korsgaard, *The Constitution of Agency* (2008, 3–5). She notes that it is a modified version of the account in her book *The Sources of Normativity* (1996, 92–94). It is of special relevance here because it describes in a particularly instructive way how there can be degrees of agency, ranged along a scale from instinctive normative perceptions to explicit, reflective, practical deliberations.

They are persons, but the abilities they lack mean that they, like many other animals, may face a human social world unwilling or unable to accommodate this form of agency in ways that keep it healthy.

Simple rational agency. It appears from the anthropological and historical record that the human social world from the arrival of *Homo sapiens* onward has typically been arranged to accommodate well (and without raising questions of basic justice) only those people who achieve the complex forms of self-consciousness, memory, imagination, deliberation, and choice that define at least a simple form of rational agency. This form of agency comes through the acquisition of spoken language by human beings with personal animal agency, and their consequent ability to represent themselves, to themselves, as persons with a history that might be explained, and an understanding of the world that can be summarized for practical purposes, and an awareness of the range of their goal-directed activities that can be projected as a coherent short-term plan for the future. This form of simple rational agency is characteristic of healthy human children by the age, perhaps, of four or five. And most human societies are organized to accommodate it and spend a good deal of effort helping children develop it further. There are, however, considerable differences from society to society in how much further they expect, or want, such rational agency to develop.

Complex rational agency; simple moral agency. Large, organized societies typically expect more than that—not only rational agency *simpliciter*, but a more developed form of it (moral agency). This comes through the development of a complex, reflective personality, of significant deliberative powers, with the ability to translate all of that into choice, decision, and action in pursuit of long-range goals, and of the disposition to accept causal responsibility for such actions. In modern social environments, it usually also involves fluency with a written language and extensive education through its use.

The point is not simply that there is great variation across our species in the extent to which we become agents. The point is also that a theory of basic justice will have to deal with that full range of human beings. As a matter of consistency, it will presumably also have to deal with all other comparable agents of whatever species.

2.2. *The robustness of the developmental track toward complex rational agency*

It is important to pay attention to the fact that human neurophysiology (even when it is quite far outside the range of the typical) is set up to drive development persistently toward complex forms of agency—toward lives whose waking moments are characterized by self-aware, effective, goal-directed activity—activity that is responsive to information we acquire about our environments when it is especially relevant to achieving those goals.

Think of what deprivations it would take to ensure that a human infant lacked the necessary physical endowments for that sort of development; or to ensure that a human infant who *had* those endowments nonetheless *could not* develop complex rational agency. Think of the extent of disease or injury necessary to prevent it. The point is that this developmental track for human beings—from rudimentary animal agency to complex forms of rational agency—is quite robust. Such agency develops with even minimally good physical and psychological health, in any minimally favorable physical and social environment.

Self-habilitation. Once acquired, such complex rational agency becomes a relentless source of self-habilitation. It can go badly wrong in the sense of becoming self-defeating—as in cases of learned helplessness. But it can also go very well in the sense of dramatically reducing the need for direct habilitative efforts from others. And the coping abilities we acquire through the exercise of our agency are often powerful sources of self-sustaining levels of physical and psychological health—even for people who begin with, or acquire, significant disabilities of other sorts. Robustly healthy agents often need help from others, and even with such help, are all too obviously mortal. But that does nothing to undermine the way in which agency can make the most of even the most impoverished set of endowments—and the most challenging health conditions and environments in which we can survive.

The necessity of complex rational agency for the development of moral agency. It is also clear that much of the habilitation required to go beyond the point of simple rational agency—to become the moral agents addressed by theories of justice—*cannot* be directly supplied by others. This point is as old as Aristotle's answer to the question of whether virtue can be taught. He observed that many things that cannot be taught can nonetheless be learned. And it is a short step from that to identifying a large class of things—most of them having to do with the development of moral agency—which must be *self*-supplied in an important sense. What others can do is provide favorable circumstances in which agents can learn to take the initiative, learn to be persistent, and learn the other traits of active, effective agency. But unless the agents themselves practice these things on their own, so to speak, such traits do not develop beyond rudimentary, fragile impulses.

3. Good (Basic) Health as Reliably Competent Functioning

Health is about physical and psychological functioning, over the complete range of levels from worst-possible to best-possible. Basic health covers the fundamental layer of that, from worst-possible to basically good health. Defined in terms of physical and psychological functioning, good health at the basic level may be characterized as *reliably competent functioning in a given range of environments.* If the functioning is less than competent, or less than reliable (in strength and stability), it is less than good health. If it is more than merely competent, or more than merely reliable in strength and stability, it is more than merely good.

Much of this competent functioning is at the autonomic level: physiological processes in all major organ systems. This includes the neurophysiological sources of the energy and motivation for activity that are sensitive to environmental variables, including primal impulses, goal-directedness, and intention. It also includes a wide array of similar psychological processes—both unconscious and conscious—all of it ultimately connected to the coping activity characteristic of human agents. And it is interesting to note that all these processes, from the most minute biochemical ones to the most elaborate forms of self-conscious deliberation, choice, and action can be illuminated by analogy to feedback mechanisms that adjust physical and psychological processes with respect to environmental "disturbances" (Landreth, 2009). Some of these processes are homeostatic; others are generative, developmental, or progressive.

3.1. *Environmental diversity and required functioning*

Competent functioning in a given environment is by definition adequate for that environment; it meets requirements. Some environments are not survivable for human beings; what they require is beyond what human endowments and habilitative efforts can achieve or sustain. This illustrates starkly that the possibilities for habilitation toward good health are determined by the intersection of human endowments (including their developmental momentum and heterogeneous motivational elements) and the demands imposed by surrounding physical and social environments.

Those environments are diverse, both in scale and content. People competent to function in one range of them (say, in rural agricultural environments in a wide range of cultures) may find themselves poorly equipped even to survive in others. Some unsurvivable environments can be escaped, of course, or habilitated into minimally or genuinely hospitable ones. But it is obvious that many human beings who function competently in a large, postindustrial society would not be able to do so in a small-scale society functioning with stone tools, or to do the long-term, physically demanding work required to habilitate a barely survivable physical environment on a frontier into a more hospitable one. Such an environment puts a premium on physiological health and strength—as well as strength in those aspects of agency that involve practical intelligence of a survivalist sort, resourcefulness, persistence, courage, and endurance. It puts a premium on social usefulness for physical survival—including the level of communicative and empathic abilities, along with the level of trustworthiness, cooperation, and conviviality necessary for a minimally hospitable social environment. It may have little initial use for the ability to read or write, or for science (as opposed to engineering), or for philosophy (as opposed to cosmology and religion), or for politics, law, or ethics (as opposed to tribal identity, customs, and settled conventions for adapting to changed circumstances), or for art (as opposed to education and entertainment). Diabetics would not survive for long. Neither would those who suffer spinal cord injuries. And philosophers would find it hard to find a niche if, for example, they happen also to be equipped with fragile psyches and an aversion to physical labor.

All of this illustrates the same point: what counts as reliably competent functioning—that is, what counts as good health—differs dramatically from one physical and social environment to another. An environment defines necessities for individual and social survival, just as human physical and psychological endowments do. And we should add that human beings who function competently in one environment very often function competently in a range of closely related ones, since the list of necessities in each of them overlaps greatly. Moreover, some human beings function competently in a large range of quite diverse environments: they have capabilities necessary for life in a stone age material culture, and for a life in academia. Think of an anthropologist who is able to do fieldwork for some years without recourse to a modern medical kit or modern survival tools. It is true also for explorers, merchants, or soldiers fit enough, and talented enough, to survive and thrive in a wide range of environments.

This has consequences for basic justice if good health is one of its goals. A conception of good health will have to be sensitive to the range of environments in which an individual can reliably function competently, both physiologically and psychologically. And it seems plausible to think that any conception of good health should imply reliably competent physiological and psychological functioning in at least a range of closely related environments. But the question is how wide the range should be.

Part of the answer comes from considering the range of difficulties people can reasonably be expected to face throughout their lives, and the sort of health they would need in order to cope with those difficulties. Some of those difficulties come from injuries, diseases, and other forms of ill health that occur within a given environment. Others come from changes in the environment itself, or from moving into or out of a given environment. Life in ancient Greece and Rome, for example, included general vulnerability to major shifts in social status: enslavement as a result of capture during war; exile, sometimes including loss of property and citizenship, and consequent vulnerability to enslavement, or to a solitary, miserable existence; subjection to the whims of tyrants; and so forth. And in every society that is subject to wars or revolution or economic collapse, people are vulnerable to dramatic shifts in social status as well. Reliably competent functioning in all these societies requires considerable adaptability.

Stability, strength, and adaptability. For the purposes of connecting good health to basic justice, it seems reasonable to think of the range of environments involved in terms of the level of adaptability ordinary people might actually have to have in order to thrive throughout their lifetimes. What difficulties are they likely to face within their initial environments? What changes in those initial environments are likely? What is the likelihood that they will have to leave an environment they inhabit and move into another one for which they have not been habilitated?

The general problem raised by this set of questions is one of identifying the appropriate balance between stability, strength, and adaptability—the balance appropriate for good health as a goal for basic justice. The problem is that habilitation for any given environment is likely to produce forms of strength and stability in behavioral dispositions—and in the functioning of agency—and that make it difficult or even impossible for individuals to adapt to forced changes.

Sometimes these difficulties come from intense attachments that fasten the individual to a particular form of life. History and literature are full of stories of people who are unable to reconcile themselves to the loss of a child, or a spouse, or a career, or honor, or pride in their work, or the way things used to be. We understand some of these difficulties as a necessary consequence of good health, of appropriate forms of its strength and stability, since they indicate the presence of attachments and loves and hopes and sources of sustained joy that are part of a flourishing life. But we also understand that there are pathological forms of rigidity—for example, in attachment, love, pride, and grief.

Such behavioral rigidity sometimes comes from habitual epistemic expectations and routines that are very reliable and effective in one environment but are unreliable or even lethal in another. Sometimes it comes from difficulties in learning a second or third or fourth language, or a particular new language. Sometimes it comes from developing specialized abilities incompatible with those required by another environment (competent warriors unable to function well when they come home). We understand some of these difficulties, also, as a consequence of good health—as predictable forms of its strength and stability in a given environment. Yet it is natural to think that there also must be pathological forms of such strength and stability, marked not by mere difficulty in adapting to change, but by the impossibility of it, at least in some circumstances.

Basic justice is about practicable requirements. It need not be concerned with fanciful environments that we have no reason to think human beings will ever have to inhabit or can actually be properly habilitated for. But it does have very good reason to be concerned with the adaptability that foreseeable circumstances might require of people, both ordinary and extraordinary ones. So the question of the appropriate balance between strength, stability, and adaptability will be answered not only in terms of what is likely to be needed but also in terms of what can be practicably provided by (re)habilitation.

3.2. *Developmental stage variance*

The health scale developed in Chapter 5 will show how a conception of good health can be defined so as to accommodate these concerns about adaptability and to specify the range of environments involved in an ascription of good health. It will also make clear that such ascriptions also require an appropriate adjustment for the individual's age, or more precisely, the person's position on an expected developmental trajectory. That developmental trajectory is determined by beginning with the trajectory that is the statistical norm in a given environment and then adjusting for the individual's initial physiological endowments, and any additional, permanent impairments.

Agency and the coherent or integrated personality. It will turn out that good health will involve considerable integration of the heterogeneous factors of human personality—their integration into a coherent motivational and behavioral structure. And it will turn out that the powers of complex rational agency are needed to provide that sort of integration. It is those powers, and the forms of integration resulting from them, which generate the dispositions about justice discussed later.

3.3. *Hospitable environments*

As noted earlier, what counts as good health varies significantly from one environment to another because the necessary habilitative tasks and coping abilities in them can differ dramatically. It does not follow, however, that every aspect of good basic health varies in this way. And the aspect of basic health at issue in this part of the argument is its behavioral competency in a given range of environments— that is, the behavioral drives, dispositions, tendencies, and coping abilities that characterize basically healthy agency in those environments. It is there, if anywhere in healthy functioning, that we will find analogs to the norms of basic justice.

If the object is to match up basic health with basic justice, however, it is reasonable to work with the same overall range of environments in both cases. If the norms of basic justice apply only in a limited range of environments—or if those norms apply differently in different ranges—we should look for similar limitations or differences in basically healthy agency.

Healthy agency in hospitable environments. Paying attention to the circumstances of habilitation suggests that the fundamental motivational structure and capabilities of healthy agency might be quite constant across all genuinely hospitable environments.[2] And it is possible that this constancy extends as well to those survivable or minimally hospitable environments which can be habilitated into something genuinely hospitable. Efforts at such habilitation would be strongly motivated for healthy agents and would be aimed at the same fundamental goals as those involved in sustaining genuinely hospitable environments.

Below the threshold of potentially hospitable environments, however, things are as problematic for basic health as they are for basic justice. Good health is certainly not possible for long in an environment that is not survivable, and theories of justice differ in their expectations about basic justice in such circumstances. Similarly, a Hobbesian state of nature incapable of habilitation into something healthier is also incapable of habilitation into something resembling basic justice.

So it seems right to examine the conception of basic health across all hospitable, and potentially hospitable, environments. If there is no significant convergence in the motivational structure and capabilities of healthy agency across the full range of such environments, then the conception of basic health will be too environment-relative to match up with the conception of basic justice.

---

[2] In the discussion of the circumstances of habilitation, the notion of a genuinely hospitable environment was defined as one in which succeeding generations of human beings living in communities regularly flourish in good health for long periods. This does not restrict such environments to those stable enough to persist for a century, or even half that long. But it does exclude environments that are merely survivable for groups or isolated individuals for short periods, when their efforts are solely devoted to their own survival and not that of succeeding generations. And it also excludes environments that are merely minimally hospitable ones in which people can survive for longer periods, with some time and energy to spend on things other than survival but without the sort of social stability that permits successful multigenerational habilitation.

5

Robustly Healthy Agency

As noted earlier, the general concept of health that frames this discussion is one that is commonly employed in contemporary medical, psychiatric, and psychological *practice*—even if it may be incautiously elided in textbook and mission-statement definitions of health. This concept assumes that the notion of health properly ranges over various levels of both ill health and good health. But it also assumes that health does not extend all the way out to "perfect" health. Rather, it confines itself to the region in which there are significant, two-way causal and conceptual connections between positive and negative health. The assumption is that while functionally significant levels of ill health compromise or at least threaten all levels above them, the reverse is not true beyond a certain level of robustness: a life bereft of bliss or significantly short of perfection does not necessarily drive us toward ill health.

This practical concept of health is naturalistic, individualistic, functional, and environmentally situated: health refers to "significant" matters of physiological and psychological functioning, for given individuals, in a given set of environments. This means that the general concept of health used here, and analogous general concepts that are at least implicit in much contemporary research and practice in health science, are unified and limited versions of a concept of health traceable to the eudaimonistic tradition:

The health of an individual human being is a set of functionally significant traits and/or states defined on a range running from nonsurvivable forms of disease, deficit, disorder, impairment, injury, or distress (ill health) to states or traits of physical or psychological strength, resistance, resilience, momentum, energy and activity (good health) that have reciprocal causal connections to ill health.

I will argue that this general concept, with some elaboration to be given later, makes it possible to see how we might eventually work out a full-fledged conception of health that has two properties of particular interest to normative theories of justice: it can resolve the indexing problem for normative theories of basic justice, and it is comprehensive enough to function as the representative good in such theories.

The first part of this elaboration concerns the use of health as a metric to solve the indexing problem *for health*. That will be addressed in this chapter. The second part (about health as the representative good for theories of justice) addresses the indexing problem for basic justice generally. It will be addressed in the next chapter.

1. The Health Metric

1.1. *Traits and conditions*

In the literature on both negative and positive health it is common to distinguish health as a trait from health as a condition, along the lines discussed in Chapter 3. It is not a contradiction for a physician to write something like this: "Healthy adult female, sleep deprived due to overwork, presenting with an upper respiratory infection and fever." Or "Healthy adult male facing a tenure decision, presenting with generalized anxiety and specific worries about his erratic behavior at department meetings." The term "healthy" in those phrases refers to health as a trait—in particular, to a finding that the patients have a range of important capabilities for rehabilitation which can be expected to move them away from their unhealthy conditions, given relatively modest interventions, and back into a stable condition in which the infection and fever, or the anxiety, are absent.

People who are healthy in this trait sense can suddenly develop conditions that are quite serious—even lethal if left untreated. But the capacity for habilitation or rehabilitation is crucial to the trait/condition distinction. Only if people develop unhealthy conditions that are, or are at risk of being, seriously resistant to habilitation or rehabilitation do we revise our *trait* assessment from healthy to unhealthy.

We can think of the trait of health, then, as various degrees of vitality beginning at a state just discernibly above death and rising in increments through various age-adjusted levels of bad health, good health, and excellent health to terminate in optimal health of indefinite duration. What we need for present purposes is a rough identification of the physiological, psychological, and environmental factors of vitality that, taken together, constitute the capacity for habilitation and rehabilitation—both away from unhealthy conditions and toward restored or improved health traits.

Health professionals make such assessments routinely, though more or less piecemeal—in triage, in emergency or intensive care settings, in hospital admissions or discharge processes, in medical or psychological rehabilitation settings, and so forth. The judgments that come out of such assessments address the possibilities for restorative, ameliorative, or palliative therapies. I say these routine decisions are often piecemeal because they often focus on only part of the health equation: physical as opposed to psychological factors, or the reverse, or either of those without careful consideration of the family setting or larger environment.

1.2. *Capacities for habilitation and rehabilitation: An illustration*

The task here is to try to put all of those well-recognized factors together in the context of habilitation. Ultimately, this will require turning the general concept of health into a detailed, full-fledged conception of it. That is a task for philosophically sophisticated people in the health sciences—in research, public health, and clinical practice.

What I will do here is merely to illustrate how such a full-fledged conception of health might be organized, and how its metric could be useful for normative theories of justice. This illustration will be an appropriate beginning if it identifies capacities that are routinely assessed with some precision in the health sciences. That means expressing them in terms that are as independent of ethical theory and cultural norms as, say, norms about minimum daily standards for nutrition. The following outline is intended to meet those conditions in a preliminary way and to cover the range of issues raised by the general concept of health defined earlier.

Factors of trait-health. We begin by taking individuals as we find them: each with a given set of physical and psychological endowments, in a given social and natural environment, and with a given set of health *conditions,* negative or positive. We then focus on their health traits—their capacities for habilitation and rehabilitation.

Consider the following general factors of trait-health, as they might occur on both the negative and positive sides of the health spectrum. All these factors summarize capacities for habilitation and rehabilitation, measured in terms of physical and psychological functioning.

a. *Resistance* to declines toward ill health, in traits or conditions. Such resistance may operate against declines that are entirely within the categories of good or ill health, or against declines that take us from good health into ill health. One's immune system is an example of resistance (or lack of it) in this sense. So is physiological or psychological strength in various other organic or behavioral systems.

b. *Resilience,* via homeostatic mechanisms, in returning to a previous level of health from a lesser level. As in the case of resistance, resilience may operate entirely within the categories of good or ill health, or across those categories. Cardiopulmonary functioning with respect to blood gases is an example of homeostatic resilience (or lack of it) in this sense. Psychological defense mechanisms of various sorts are also examples of homeostatic resilience.

c. *Restorative capacities* that can, under some habilitative conditions, reverse the declines toward ill health that occur despite an individual's resistance or resilience, or can repair damage to the mechanisms of resistance and resilience themselves. Example: in some cases of acute kidney failure, in which homeostatic mechanisms of resilience have been defeated, kidneys retain the capacity to restore their functioning if they are properly rested temporarily with dialysis. On the psychological side, rest, recreation, and diversions of various sorts can have a restorative effect. And regenerative physical and psychological processes are also part of these restorative capacities.

d. *Generation of agent-energy*—that is, generation of the sort of physical and psychological energy necessary for initiating and sustaining goal directed activity. Lethargy is the absence of such energy, whose levels are sensitive to many things, including blood gases, drugs, depression, optimism, stress, and nutrition.

e. *Generation of momentum for development toward good health* (physical, cognitive, emotional, and conative) along its developmental track over a complete life. Factors that supply such momentum include agent-energy, stimulating, stable environments that reinforce exploratory activity, and the emulation of developmental models. Obvious examples of physical factors that impede this are permanent or lasting impairments such as traumatic brain injuries, the loss of limbs, or paralysis. Examples of impeding psychological factors are psychogenic learning disorders, or disruptive emotional disorders.

f. *Generation of the self-initiated activity characteristic of good health* along its developmental track over a complete life. Passivity is the absence of this factor of good health, which is in general the failure to translate energy and momentum into effective, self-initiated activity. Examples of physical sources of this problem are certain brain injuries that make it impossible for people to formulate preferences about various options and formulate plans about the future. On the psychological side, examples include various patterns of behavior in which initiative and self-command have been limited or extinguished.

The three "R" factors (a, b, c) address the problem of stabilizing a given level of physiological and psychological health with respect to declines, leaving it open or labile with respect to improvements. The three "G" factors (d, e, f) address the energy, momentum, scope, and direction of the capability for habilitation and rehabilitation toward improved physical and psychological health. But all six of these factors are elements of that capability.

Dimensions of variance. Further, we can plausibly assume that each of the six factors varies along the same three dimensions: *the range of environments* (E) in which they are operative; *the range of health conditions* (C) with respect to which they are operative; and their operative *strength* (S).

We can think of strength as the degree of resistance to change or momentum toward it around a given point on the vitality continuum. What is built into the notion of health is the notion of an *optimal* level of resistance and momentum.

Optimal resistance to declines gives us optimal security against reversals at each point. Optimal momentum toward improvements gives us optimal possibilities for habilitation or rehabilitation. To say that a factor is at zero strength is to say that it has no resistance to declines, and no momentum toward improvements.

Incapability is the zero point for each factor along each dimension. Absent arguments to the contrary, more of each factor along each dimension is preferable—healthier—than less. So, as long as we work only with these factors or others like them, it should be possible to define an intelligible scale, for the purposes of public policy, ranging from the worst form of health to the best (or at least the best that is of practical importance), and ultimately to distinguish the worst-off members of society (in terms of health) from those in various strata above them.

1.3. *A note on mathematical representation*

We want to represent health as a set of six health factors (a, b, c, d, e, f), measured along each of three dimensions, strength, environments, and *trait*-health conditions (S, E, C), minus the deformations in that measurement caused by Transient-health conditions (T). So we imagine, first, that there is a separate scoring system in each dimension for each of the six factors, and a scoring system as well, in positive numbers, for transient-health conditions within each dimension as a whole (T_S, T_E, T_C), or with respect to individual traits in those dimensions T_{sa}, T_{ea}, T_{ca} . . .

We then assume that each scoring system will yield trait by trait numerical values which can be manipulated to achieve a composite score for each dimension. The conjunction of those composite scores is a representation of a particular "health state" that implicitly defines a particular level of trait-functioning.

$$\text{Health state } X_n = (S - T_S)_n + (E - T_E)_n + (C - T_C)_n$$

Any health state X_n can thus be represented in a three-dimensional graph with S, E, and C as the axes, where the volume is adjusted appropriately by the value of T for each axis. A series of such graphs can be used to represent changes toward or away from some baseline health state. However, such graphic representation obscures the values for each trait, as well as the extent to which transient health conditions (T) are initially reflected in each trait's functioning.

To keep those values distinct, we may represent each dimension (S, E, C) as a column vector of the health trait-values marked with their burden of transient health conditions, running from zero upward. These column vectors will yield a health state matrix that can give a much more detailed representation of the health state than that given by the three-dimensional graphs.

$$\begin{pmatrix} S_{a\text{-}Tsa} & E_{a\text{-}Tea} & C_{a\text{-}Tca} \\ S_{b\text{-}Tsb} & E_{b\text{-}Teb} & C_{b\text{-}Tcb} \\ S_{c\text{-}Tsc} & E_{c\text{-}Tec} & C_{c\text{-}Tcc} \\ S_{d\text{-}Tsd} & E_{d\text{-}Ted} & C_{d\text{-}Tcd} \\ S_{e\text{-}Tse} & E_{e\text{-}Tee} & C_{e\text{-}Tce} \\ S_{f\text{-}Tsf} & E_{f\text{-}Tef} & C_{f\text{-}Tcf} \end{pmatrix}$$

Sequences of such matrices can also be used to represent (and calculate the probabilities of) change from one state to another. Setting up the matrices will sometimes be tedious, since a substantial transition matrix (e.g., 6 × 6 or 18 × 18 depending on the level of detail one wants to track) will be needed to calculate changes from one health state to another, and since the range of values that the variables can take will often have to be managed for computational purposes. (For example, in Markov chains each column sums to 1; other methods exist that may be more flexible.) Applications of linear algebra apparently have the resources to make such tedium not only possible but rewarding—not to mention that computers can make the actual computations themselves painless, or at least not a detriment to the health of public policy analysts.[1]

1.4. *The health scale*

Worst health. Suppose, no doubt contrary to fact, that this list of factors is exhaustive. Then the worst form of trait-health will be the one in which all these factors are at zero along each dimension. The person lacks (a. . . . f) completely, with respect to every health condition to which he or she might be subject, in every accessible environment. It is the point of least resistance to unhealthy conditions, and the point of least resilience from them. It is the point of least restorative power, momentum, energy, and activity for habilitation. Examples of people with the worst possible health are difficult to find—presumably because they are very, very near death—so near that even identifying that state eludes a clinician.

The next worst-off form of trait-health will be the one in which only one of these factors is above zero, but is just discernibly above zero, with respect to only one unhealthy condition, and is effective in only one accessible environment. And so we progress incrementally up the scale of vitality, giving whatever weights to individual factors are necessary to represent clinical realities.

Worst-off members of society (in terms of health). For the purposes of habilitation and rehabilitation, however, we cannot simply identify the worst-off members of society as all and only those with the worst form of trait-health. Vitality is not only

---

[1] Thanks to Caren Diefenderfer for steering my reflections on these matters.

a product of traits; it is also a product of occurrent ("transient"), health-related conditions. So the worst-off category will be those whose *overall* health score is lowest, where that score represents the level of trait-health *including* occurrent conditions of ill health (diseases, injuries, environmental limitations, etc.). There are thus many combinations of health conditions and health-traits that for purposes of public policy can be grouped together in the category of the worst off.

Better health. We can use the same six factors, along the same three dimensions, to describe various levels of better health—and correspondingly better off members of society. We can do this by describing levels at which the strength of various factors is increased, or the range of environments widened, or the level of treatment required for recovery from certain conditions is lessened.

Good health* and robust health. The general idea is to move upward until we find a level of health (call it robust health) at which all the factors are stable and strong in a wide range of environments, with respect to a wide variety of ordinary health conditions, given merely competent habilitation of the sorts available in those environments. This is something better than merely good health, which is a term we often use with an asterisk, indicating a significant limitation of some sort—perhaps that a change of environment or a change in daily routine will reveal serious deficiencies in trait-health.

Someone who is ventilator dependent, for example, will sometimes be described as being in good health (with an implicit asterisk), meaning that she has a good immune system, stable organ function, and no life-threatening conditions at the moment. But the asterisk reminds us that a widespread natural disaster or a war that interrupts the supply of electricity will immediately reveal a lethal deficiency in trait-health—a deficiency in the range of environments in which survival is possible.

Robust health is the level at which we typically remove the asterisks—at least the ones related to the capacity for habilitation. It is the level at which we do not attribute ordinary illnesses, diseases, or injuries to deficiencies in trait-health.

2. Health Science: Limited and Unified

2.1. *Relation to ethical theory*

Notice that this general concept of health makes no direct reference to subjective well-being, positive hedonic states, life-satisfaction, or purely psychological happiness. It looks as though it might not be predictable, at least for individual cases, whether subjects would report such things if they have good health along the lines just described. Some people are generally buoyant, optimistic, and happy with what they have even when they have very little. Others are generally dour, pessimistic, and unhappy about what they lack, even when they have a great deal. As noted in Chapter 3.3, there is more than anecdotal evidence linking subjective well-being to good health—to agent-energy and purposive action, for example. If that is so, a lack of such well-being would show up in the scoring of various factors and reduce the overall health scores. It is less clear to me what we can predict about self-reported subjective well-being by knowing a person's overall health score—or for that matter, what we can predict about populations on that basis. A full-fledged conception of health would presumably work out these connections. But it seems plausible to withhold judgment here, so as not to rule out, pretheoretically, a conception of health in which a tragic or pessimistic view of life is compatible with robust health.

Moreover, this general concept does not make direct reference to moralized traits (moral virtues), or to the relation between health and one's ultimate aim or conception of a good life. As noted earlier, healthy human development is necessarily connected to the development of traits that overlap significantly with moral virtues. Sociality, courage, and practical wisdom are examples. But this general concept of health is cast (or at least is intended to be cast) in terms of traits that can be studied empirically and that are independent of competing conceptions of the highest good(s) as those conceptions are described in ethical theories. It would be possible, for example, for a theologian to argue, without challenging anything in the *general* definition of health or a full-fledged conception developed from it, that progress beyond good health is an unimportant good, compared to following God's law. It would similarly be possible for a philosopher to argue that while health is an important good, a direct concern for one's subjective well-being is ignoble. It would not be possible for an ethical theorist to argue that nihilism was healthy, or that slavery was healthy for slaves, or that the subordination of women was healthy for women. But then, it is presumably not an essential part of the effort to justify nihilism or slavery or the subordination of women that those practices are healthy for their victims.

2.2. *Relation to health science*

If a general concept like this works, it will define criteria of relevance, completeness, accuracy, and utility for assessing and reorganizing the many features of health discussed in the health sciences, including the science of positive health. It is meant to define a piece of terrain, barren of normative theories of justice, about which such normative theories can be constructed.

But this illustrative general concept is also meant to be modestly useful for health science itself in a number of ways. The terms used within it (stability, resilience, regeneration, generation, agent energy, and so forth) are meant to preserve the close connections between physiology and psychology often found there.

Moreover, it shows that developing a full-fledged conception of health along these lines would involve empirical work of a substantial sort.

That work would have to test hypotheses about (1) what physical and psychological equipment is necessary to achieve and sustain each general level of health; (2) what mechanisms move us from minimal ill health to good to excellent to ideal health; (3) to what extent normal development and maturation alone can drive such movement under favorable conditions; (4) what physical and psychological traits and levels of strength best drive such movement under various conditions, and which ones best support each stage in which environments; (5) whether, and under what conditions, movement from one stage to another is likely to be preferred by subjects, and movement toward it subjectively motivated; (6) how and under what conditions subjective well-being is implicated and expressed in each stage, and implicated in movement from one stage to another. And so on. It defines a substantial research agenda for empirical work that enlarges the ones that are reflected in the mission statements of some research organizations and funding sources.

3. Habilitation into Robustly Healthy Agency

Robust health, for human beings, necessarily includes robustly healthy agency. There is a conceptual connection—an expectation based on our understanding of human nature—that good health, and in particular robustly good health, will always include a comparably robust level of agency, adjusted for the individual's developmental stage. (The sort of agency found in a robustly healthy human infant is of course different from that found in a similarly healthy child, adolescent, adult, and elderly human being. The human organism, in the species-typical course of a complete life, has a substantially different constitution, physically and psychologically, at different major developmental stages.)

This connection between health and healthy agency is functional as well as conceptual. Without robustly healthy agency, one lacks abilities necessary for the self-monitored and self-initiated activity often involved with sustaining other elements of health at a robust level. The necessity for recognizing and accommodating oneself to significant changes in one's social or physical environment shows this in a pointed way, but there are many subtle, everyday ways in which impaired agency damages health generally. So threats or damage to agency are by that fact also threats or damage to some other areas of robust health. Brain-injured adults who have lost the ability to make new memories, to have preferences long enough to make plans and consequently to make choices and construct lives for themselves are massively impaired with respect to healthy adult functioning of many sorts related to the activities of daily living—even if they are reasonably healthy otherwise, physically and psychologically (Damasio, 1999, 43–47, 113–21).

The reverse is not quite true. Ill health often has consequences for the health of one's agency in the activities of daily living, but this is not always the case—especially when we consider how well people with chronic diseases or disabilities may function in a favorable environment. Type 1 diabetes, for example, is a serious health condition, but it does not necessarily compromise healthy agency in environments in which insulin and other elements of effective therapy are accessible and properly employed by the diabetic. If one's agency is unhealthy to begin with, however, or is compromised by some other health condition (brain injury, alcoholism, relentless social oppression), diabetes becomes a much larger health problem—perhaps even a lethal one.

This close conceptual and functional connection between robust health and robustly healthy agency is understandably reflected also in what aspects of health people typically care most about preserving. The loss of adult forms of complex rational agency—that is, the mental aspects of one's adult personhood, including memory, anticipation, intention, planning, and the ability to be the author of one's own life—is typically much more dreadful to contemplate than the loss of physical abilities, when the social and physical environment allows the two things to be separated. (In extreme circumstances, they might not be separable. In a slave labor camp or in the Antarctic, a broken femur may lead to death so swiftly that the idea of a preference for agency over the loss of a leg may be nonsensical.)

3.1. *Robust health as an upper boundary for basic justice*

Nonetheless, robust health and the agency it includes define an important boundary for theories of justice. Above that boundary, up through the territory of well-being toward the vanishing point of perfect happiness and virtue, comparably improved health does not seem to play a necessary role in a conception of *basic* justice. This is so because beyond the level of robust health, further improvements in well-being seem supererogatory for individuals—more than we can reasonably require of them and effectively enforce, and more than we need to concern ourselves with in designing social institutions. (In fact, robust health itself is a good deal more than any reasonably just society can expect to achieve for all of its citizens—even those with the appropriate natural endowments who are living in favorable circumstances. Chance plays too large a role in these health matters for us to expect success along these lines. But that is true of basic justice generally. And it is good that our aspirations exceed our grasp from time to time.)

Further, failing to achieve more than robust health does not seem to be a predictor of further decline toward ill health—since that level of health will include active, effective agency *sustained by relevant features of the social, political, and physical environment*, and it will be characteristic of robust psychological health in that it can cope with a failure to achieve more along the road to perfect well-being. We can certainly continue the analogy between health and happiness all the way out to perfect well-being and virtue by thinking of levels of health, fitness, and physical or psychological virtuosity that lie beyond robust health. But it becomes increasingly difficult to find *reciprocal* causal connections between those very high levels of health and the ones below them. Robust health may be a necessary condition for achieving even greater fitness or virtuosity; in that sense, there is a one-way causal connection between the two. But it does not follow that failing to reach those higher levels will necessarily compromise, or make vulnerable, any underlying lower level of health, from robust health downward. Failure to achieve good health* (with the asterisk), however, and then failure to remove the asterisk by achieving some measure of robust health does compromise, or at least threaten to compromise, lower levels of health.

It seems fair to say, then, that failing to rise beyond robust health does not constitute a danger that might make it a concern for basic justice. It does not yield a sufficient basis for requiring more of ourselves, or ourselves and others, by way of social intervention and assistance. That does not mean we should be indifferent to such striving, or admire it, or engage in it ourselves. It simply means it lies beyond the subject matter of basic justice. (This is true, at least, under the Aristotelian concept of "particular" justice we are using here, as opposed to a Platonic concept of "universal" justice which identifies it with virtue generally. People operating with the Platonic concept of justice might think such social intervention and assistance is required for anyone who falls short of the highest possible sort of righteousness or virtue.)

3.2. *Robustly healthy agency as a marker of adequate health generally*

As a practical matter, we can use robustly healthy agency as a presumptive measure for deciding what levels of health should get scrutiny as a matter of basic justice. Its boundaries are unclear at the level of this general concept of health, and it is natural to think that different normative theories of justice, focusing on different environments with different resources, will target different levels of it. But the point is that these disagreements are all representable by reference to levels of health from worst to robust. And since robustly healthy agency is a necessary condition for robust health generally, and captures the element of it about which we are most concerned, perhaps we can conveniently use robustly healthy agency as a presumptive marker of robust health generally—subject to some exceptions around the margins.

Consider the way in which we often decide whether a given health condition "requires" attention. We do this by making a threat assessment with respect to what we regard as centrally significant abilities and capabilities—centrally important forms of functioning. Healthy agency, in every age-adjusted developmental form throughout our lives, is significant in this way. And in fact we routinely make threat assessments about health conditions by considering impacts on it.

Examples: think about dental treatments to make healthy teeth blindingly white. Or tattoo removal, or hair removal by electrolysis. None of these is ordinarily a treatment for ill health, as defined here. They are improvements on the good health side of the ledger that people sometimes regard as important and even necessary. And it is not hard to find circumstances in which such things do influence a person's job opportunities and/or social relationships, and perhaps then, if left untreated, begin to have a seriously dysfunctional, depressive effect.

Absent significant consequences like those, we tend to exclude such matters from health, or at least from matters of basic justice concerning health. And even in the presence of those significant consequences, it is an open question as to whether the problem should be addressed by working to change social or legal norms about equal opportunity and discrimination, or by trying to strengthen the ability of the individual (the health of the person's agency) to resist depression, or to resist the cosmetic procedure, or perhaps to resist both. But notice that the question of justice here can be raised in terms of the consequences for healthy agency, and the philosophical discussion of it can be carried out largely in those terms as well. Once the consequences for agency in this case have been resolved, the issue about justice and health care seems to have been resolved also.

Similarly for health conditions that are currently asymptomatic, inconsequential for functioning, likely to remain benign, and even in the worst-case scenario are likely to become malign only very gradually, in ways that can be diagnosed and treated effectively when that happens. We can imagine cases in which some asymptomatic conditions like that are so worrisome to people that their otherwise robust agency is threatened or damaged by lack of access to the treatment. But without such a functional threat or damage to agency, it is hard to imagine that we would regard such conditions as raising matters of basic justice if treatment for them is postponed, and replaced by watchful waiting. (Think of a small nodule on an eighty-year-old man's prostate.) When such a functional threat or damage to agency arises, however, we can imagine that in some of those cases it would be better, all things considered, to pursue further tests or treatments rather than trying to make the person's psychology robust enough to withstand the postponement. The point, again, is that the question can be raised and discussed in the context of consequences for agency—and that this seems to capture both the central issue about it, and the exceptions to our policy that we want to keep in mind.

3.3. *Robustly healthy agency as a practical target*

I suggest that robustly healthy agency is a practical target for the principles normative theories of basic justice might adopt about health. It defines a standard high
enough to satisfy any reasonable level of priority for health that a normative theory
might adopt. But it also defines a movable standard, sensitive to differences in individuals, populations, and environments, and amenable as well to different political
constitutions. Nonetheless, it is not an empty target for public policy. It does assume
that making adequate social arrangements for habilitating people into robustly
healthy agency is something every normative theory of justice should address—
either by accepting some version of this goal or offering an alternative to it. Normative theories can all address this by considering the following propositions:

The basic justice of social arrangements, with respect to human health, can be assessed
in terms of habitation into robustly healthy agency.

If such social arrangements do not do all they can reasonably be expected to do, or can
reasonably afford to do, to permit people to habilitate themselves and others into robustly
healthy agency, then those social arrangements need to be corrected to do so.

However, if such social arrangements have done all they can do to achieve those goals
with respect to health, they need not go further (in terms of basic justice) except to deal
with some special cases on the margins.

Accepting a high level of robustly healthy agency as a target would be particularly important for large, complex, highly developed liberal societies with extensive international connections. They have strong interests (economic interests,
among others) in habilitating all their citizens into active, effective, socially embedded agency in as wide an array of environments as possible, with high levels of
resistance, resilience, and energy, as well as momentum for further improvement
in all of those environments. Any theory of basic justice that wishes to be relevant
for such societies would have to take account of the importance of robust health in
them.

And more generally, a high level of robustly healthy agency and the budding
eudaimonistic virtues embedded in it would be impressive, and presumably relevant to any society that has open dealings with modern liberal societies. Along
with initiative, that level of healthy agency would include robust sociality (including norms of fairness, reciprocity, benevolence, and reliability), active and effective agency (including courage and persistence), and cooperative activity.
Lesser levels of agency will clearly be disadvantages and/or disabilities in developed societies in the liberal democratic tradition, and thus to any other society
that has open dealings with them.

But notice two things about this target for justice and public policy. First, it will
be a moving target within any given society, dependent on social resources and

circumstances. Second, it will be a moving target across societies, dependent not only on social resources and circumstances but on culture-specific social norms. What counts as robust agency in a society that is deliberately closed to the world at large and thoroughly committed to a single comprehensive ethical theory will be strikingly different from what counts as robust agency in societies open to the world.

We can perhaps assume for the moment that defining the highest level of health (optimal health) will always involve reference to a comprehensive ethical theory— one that gives an account of what levels of these factors are needed to live the best sort of life available to a human being in the full range of environments in which humans can thrive. A liberal democratic polity will presumably want a health target that is neutral with respect to such theories *where they diverge from each other*. The point at which they diverge seems to be *within the range of variance* of robustly healthy agency.

6

Healthy Agency as the Representative Good for Basic Justice

The next step in the argument appears to be an unusually large one for a single short chapter. The proposal here is to use healthy agency as a unitary way of representing all the goods that we think a normative theory of basic (distributive) justice will need to address, and to represent the extent to which a given society, or a given theory of basic justice, gets distributions right.

Taken in isolation, that proposal is startling. But previous chapters have given an elaborate context for it, and the concluding chapters in Part Four (Chapters 9–10) will address some matters that this one treats either too briefly or not at all.

1. Healthy Agency versus Wealth and Income

The historical alternatives to this use of healthy agency are the use of sociopolitical status (caste, class, civil liberties), or economic status (wealth and income, resources generally), or some combination of welfare, opportunities, and capabilities as the index. Sociopolitical and economic status or resources are *sometimes* the most plausible ways of representing where people stand with respect to all the goods we care about and that we think raise questions of justice. Specifically, they are the most plausible with regard to societies which lack elaborate social institutions that can implement complex distributive policies, and that lack material conditions—including modern medicine—which promote and sustain good health. In contemporary developed societies, opportunities and capabilities (specifically, opportunities and capabilities for well-being) may seem more appropriate within egalitarian normative theories.[1] But the argument here is that health is more appropriate at the theory-independent level.

---

[1] For some of the literature on this point, and references to a good deal more, see Arneson (1989, 1990); Cohen (1989, 1993); Roemer (1998); Daniels (1990); Dworkin (1981, parts 1 and 2); Sen (2009); Vallentyne (2002).

1.1. *Wealth and income as the representative good*

For large, complex, contemporary societies that are by historical standards affluent and characterized by considerable social mobility (whether endorsed by social and legal norms or not), using wealth and income as an index remains a default position for many theorists. The thought is that wealth and income, due to their causal connections to other elements of well-being, can be used, statistically, to identify the worst-off groups in society, the next worst-off, and so forth up the scale. This is so because there are probabilistic causal connections between the quantity (relative to others) of one's secure, fungible, and transferable economic resources and the level of one's health, personal security, political power, and accessible forms of liberty, education, employment, and leisure (again, relative to others). Those things, taken together, are also probabilistically correlated with longevity and eventually with social status as well—though in societies with strong caste, class, ethnic, or theocratic systems, such changes in social status often occur in small increments, over generations.

Normative theories of distributive justice using an economic index to well-being then decide how to arrange the distribution of economic resources so that it best promotes and sustains justice in the distribution of everything else of significance to the theory. They do not, of course, adopt distributive principles and recommend public policies that deal *only* with economic resources. Even their most libertarian varieties frame economic policies with principles prohibiting crimes against persons and property, guaranteeing the enforcement of contracts, providing for the common defense, guaranteeing some level of civil liberties for citizens, and guaranteeing that citizens can purchase (or gain through need or merit) access to education and health care. Such noneconomic principles are assumed to have positive consequences for one's position on the economic index. So no matter what form of normative theory we adopt—egalitarian or inegalitarian, libertarian or communitarian, natural rights or natural teleology, consequentialist or social contract—the full range of distributive questions can be raised and answered within these strong prior constraints on economic activity. The general idea is that by measuring our progress in achieving just distributions of economic resources, we can measure our progress in achieving justice comprehensively.

1.2. *Health as the representative good*

Now, of course, the choice of economic resources as the representative good is controversial. For one thing, an economic scale doesn't reflect common ground (among comprehensive theories of the good) about basic, intrinsic goods.[2] Thus its

---

[2] Neither does opportunity, liberty, or an unrestricted notion of capabilities. Traditional, or theocratic, or agrarian societies that are deliberately closed to alternative ways of life are also likely to limit, in some cases dramatically, the extent to which they think those things measure a good life or set standards for justice.

connections to basic justice and virtue may well be accidental, depending on the nature of the social arrangements we have or that our normative theory of justice recommends. For another thing, because an economic scale is not conceptually connected to common ground about basic intrinsic goods, it is difficult to develop an upper boundary for it that is also connected to common ground about well-being. As with the health scale, the lower boundary is clear. Unlike the health scale, the upper boundary is not so clear. (Defining an economic upper boundary by reference to how much money people actually "need"—as opposed to desire— essentially imports a noneconomic criterion into the definition.)

These controversies about the use of wealth and income as the representative good have been widely reflected in philosophical work through the history of egalitarian political philosophy in particular. These alternatives include resources generally, not just economic resources. They include opportunity; well-being; opportunity for well-being; capabilities; and a complex conception of social goods in which different distributive principles, indexed by different representative goods, govern equality in different spheres of justice (Walzer, 1983).

Some of these alternatives are fundamentally pluralistic and must work around the indexing problem in ways that introduce significant difficulty and indeterminacy into normative theory. A unitary account of a single representative good is preferable to them, simply on the grounds of determinacy and simplicity, *if it is comprehensive enough, and is connected to common ground about basic intrinsic goods.* But unitary alternatives to health, such as wealth and income, seem to be less clearly comprehensive as representative goods than robustly healthy agency.

Asymmetry in restorative power. And in the case of wealth and income at least, there is a further advantage to adopting health as the representative good. Human life is filled with reversals. The goods necessary for well-being can be lost and restored in many ways, often in ways that are unanticipated and undeserved. An appropriate representative good for basic justice should be able to reflect such changes and direct us to appropriate remedies. In this respect there is an asymmetry between health and economic resources that favors the choice of health as the representative good.

Imagine an individual with robustly healthy agency and economic resources that are enough or greater than the level needed to sustain such health. Then imagine that the individual's agency is abruptly undermined through a brain injury that damages his memory and other intellectual abilities. He has access to excellent health care through insurance that pays the complete cost of rehabilitation and long-term care if needed. But he loses his income after six months (because he is not yet ready to go back to work) and simultaneously loses a great deal of his wealth, through a collapse of the value of his holdings. This means that he will remain in a long-term care facility until either his health or his wealth is restored.

Wealth is not a good index to the situation he faces, at least in this sense: the restoration of income will not be possible until he can work, a situation that calls for improved health. The restoration of his wealth will not improve his health and therefore will not be an accurate index to his overall well-being unless and until he recovers substantial memory and other intellectual ability. Again, his agency is a better index. Even without the restoration of his wealth, the restoration of his robustly healthy agency alone would improve his situation greatly, since it would by definition include significant ability to cope with his economic losses—even in the presence of significant difficulties in regaining his lost income and wealth.

Similarly for losses of just one of these two candidates for the representative good. There is an asymmetry there also—not in every case, but in many. When an individual suffers a loss in robustly healthy agency, the obvious remedy is always to look first at the possibility of restoring that level of agency. This is so even for people whose agency is damaged by their own poor choices, or vices. Yet that is not always the situation for lost wealth—*especially* when those losses are caused by the individual's own poor choices or vices. In those cases, restoring the wealth can magnify the problem, especially if shortcomings in the health of the individual's agency remain unaddressed. So when an individual suffers a loss in wealth, the obvious remedy is sometimes to look first at improving that person's agency.

Surely the adequacy of the representative good depends on its behaving in these cases in the way that robust health behaves, and not the way that economic resources (wealth and income) behave.

2. Healthy Agency versus Pluralism

The diversity of goods creates a problem for any proposal for a unitary metric. Michael Walzer makes a particularly eloquent case against the existence of any universal medium of exchange, and he notes the way in which this cuts against both traditional egalitarian theories of justice and conventional liberal ones (Walzer, 1983, Ch. 1). I do not think this cuts against a proposal for using the health scale as a metric, however.

2.1. *The Imperial Ministry of Health*

One criticism, in the form of ridicule, is sometimes made in response to the World Health Organization's definition of health as "complete" physical, psychological, and social well-being. It is that making such health a fundamental right conjures up the specter of an overarching, overly powerful Ministry of Health, in control of all government functions.

But that is a red herring in this case. Whatever its significance may be as a criticism of the World Health Organization's definition, it has no relevance to how a single unitary criterion would have to be applied across government functions. We don't think that using wealth and income as the representative good would be likely to put the Treasury Department in command of everything else. We might say that the Office of Management and Budget has its fingers in the cost-benefit analysis done by all government departments in the executive branch, but that is just one important part of a very complex governmental structure. There is no reason to think that using a health scale as a metric for basic distributive justice would disturb government structure any more than that.

2.2. *Spheres of justice*

A much more serious challenge comes from the argument that the goods to be distributed are irreducibly plural and incommensurable, such that they cannot be arranged and measured against each other on a common scale. Walzer (1983) goes further and says that each of these major types of good has its own appropriate distributive principle, operating within its sphere. And the implication is that there is no superordinate principle or standard of measurement in terms of which the various spheres can be coordinated.

In reply we should observe, first, that there is evidently some general concept of basic justice and some general concept of value operating in the background here that makes it possible for pluralists and monists to discuss these matters with each other. Further, there is evidently some meta-theoretical concept of a unitary scale operating in the background of these discussions about whether such a scale is applicable or even possible within a given normative theory of justice. So the issue of whether a health scale, defined at the meta-theoretical level, might be a defensible unitary scale is not precluded from the outset. Nor is it precluded just because a more traditional unitary scale (wealth and income) is inadequate.

Second, we should observe that the application of the different principles pluralists might propose for different spheres of justice has to be coordinated and assessed in some way so that the principles operate together in a reasonably coherent way. We can accept value pluralism—refusing to use health or anything else as a unitary measure of everything—and still use the health scale (or some alternative to it) as an indirect coordinating principle.

For example, Walzer points out that historically, economic markets have not been considered appropriate distributive mechanisms for all goods. In every society of record we have examples of what he calls "blocked exchanges." These vary from society to society. Some societies permit marriage markets, through the buying of brides. Others do not. Some societies permit the purchase of government offices. Others (Walzer gives an elaborate example from imperial China) use a meritocratic principle, and still others an electoral principle for some offices, which includes appointment powers for lesser offices. By what standard do we assess the appropriateness of these different choices for the distribution of the same goods in different societies? One way to understand the thesis here about the health scale is to suggest how it is always implicitly involved in such assessments.

First, what should we do if we find that the use of a particular distributive principle for a given sphere of justice is unhealthy in some way for the individuals who are directly or indirectly exposed to it? It is certainly plausible to hold that this always gives us at least one reason for modifying or abandoning the use of that principle in that sphere *if it is possible to do so, given the nature of the activity involved in it.* To reject the notion that health is always relevant in this way, to every proposed distributive principle in every sphere of justice, would be to insist either that the well-being of individuals is irrelevant to basic justice or that health itself is irrelevant to well-being.

Both of those options are nonstarters. No philosophically defensible theory of basic justice *ignores* the well-being of individuals—though of course some theories ignore worldly well-being in favor of its otherworldly counterpart, and some transform concerns about individual well-being into a communitarian or aggregative process of pursuing a conception of social perfection. Even in those theories, however, individual well-being is always meant to be organically connected to social perfection, much in the way that the health of individual body parts is organically connected to the health of the whole body.

So although different normative theories will employ the health scale in different ways, for different purposes, it will always be relevant to the choice of distributive principles. And if health is always relevant to the question of basic justice in this way, by giving us a reason to reject principles that are unnecessarily unhealthy, given the sphere of justice under consideration, it will (through repeated applications) lead us toward selecting the healthiest possible principles for that sphere.

Some spheres are, by their very nature, very unhealthy. So we may think that this use of the health scale doesn't amount to much. War, for example, subjects individuals to the risk of death and many health hazards short of death. Unless war can be eliminated, it is inevitable that some individuals will die or have their health seriously compromised by combat. And goals internal to the practice of war fighting will initially define nonmoral standards for it in terms of military necessity, optimal war-fighting strategy and tactics, as well as the recruitment, training, and command of soldiers in combat. Adjusting such war fighting standards toward the healthiest possible ones is obviously important, but it hardly amounts to much unless war itself is minimized or health is somehow guaranteed in other spheres.

But that is exactly what using the health scale as the common metric for basic distributive justice will accomplish. The different distributive principles for the different spheres of justice will need to be adjusted to form a coherent system. In order to do that we will need a common frame of reference—a common scale of measurement toward a shared aim. What I am proposing here is that robustly healthy agency is such a shared aim (I don't say it is the only one), that the health scale leading up to it is a workable, commonly acknowledged scale of measurement (I don't say it is the only one), and that it is the best choice for such a representative good for normative theories of justice.

3. The Representativeness of Habilitation into Healthy Agency

Many of the reasons for proposing health as the representative good have already been given: causal connections between robustly healthy agency and all the other goods we need to distribute fairly—as a matter of basic justice—are clear and direct. I think its necessity for a good life and its status as a basic, intrinsic good is much more widely recognized than the necessity of wealth or the necessity of any other representative good that has been proposed. (That is part of what accounts for its rather uncontroversial prominence as a political goal throughout the world.) It generates a health scale that can be used to resolve the indexing problem, and that scale has a natural upper boundary, definable in terms of health itself. Furthermore, the use of robustly healthy agency as the representative good keeps us on common ground at the pretheoretical level. It does not force us out of theory-independent arguments prematurely and into reliance on ones drawn from a particular ethical or even metaphysical theory.

Nonetheless, there is still more to say about why we should accept health as the representative good, and robustly healthy agency as the target level of that good.

Constitutive aims of habilitation. Norms of habilitation into health and healthy agency are constitutive, and not merely regulatory, aims of public policy in any political system in which the well-being of at least some identifiable class of citizens is a constitutive aim. This is not necessarily the case for wealth, at least on the common ground of theory-independent considerations. Some normative theories of justice have (historically) been hostile to the acquisition of wealth and to thinking of its possession as a constitutive good. In this way, the choice of robustly healthy agency is preferable to wealth. The question is whether there are other constitutive aims for habilitation that are even more inclusive. I will leave that question aside for the moment.

Basic, intrinsic good. As mentioned earlier, healthy agency is a basic, intrinsic good. So it is not arbitrary to employ an overarching scale of priorities that is implicit in such habilitation—a scale of priorities, for example, that puts this habilitation above the provision of goods that are less basic, less durable, and less fecund for human life. In this way also it is unlike wealth, which is neither basic nor intrinsic.

Relation to diversity. Moreover, pluralistic societies with commitments to individual liberty will want to allow people to flourish under a variety of comprehensive conceptions of the good—not just every imaginable conception, but quite a variety of them. The world is pluralistic. Every open society is pluralistic. And every society engaging in extensive economic and social commerce in the world is under pressure to accommodate pluralistic populations. Egalitarian commitments, to the extent that we have them, impose a further constraint on public policy, for then when we make certain goods available to some citizens, we must make sure we do not thereby disadvantage others. The world is not egalitarian. But if such tendencies exist anywhere, they exist with respect to health.

It is therefore at least initially plausible to think that habilitation into robustly healthy agency might be as far as we can reasonably go in efforts to work out egalitarian distributive policies, even within systems committed to individual liberty. Think of the matching limits we might have in the closely related area of education: how much of it we are willing to make compulsory; how much of it beyond that compulsory level we are willing to make available to everyone at public expense; how much of it we are willing to encourage everyone to pursue, through the use of publicly funded incentives. We can plausibly conclude that those standards are included in the pursuit of robustly healthy agency.

3.1. *Relevance to other goods and sectors of society*

We need to remind ourselves in detail of the way habilitation into robust health employs all of the existing organizational structures devoted to health, education, and social welfare generally. Perhaps the easiest way to see the scale of this undertaking and how it might cover all the territory we need to cover, and only that territory, is to fix our attention on a clear picture of the apex of robustly healthy agency—in adults, in developed societies roughly like our own, who satisfy the conditions of robust health along the lines outlined here without the need for making adjustments for their ages.

Such people are by definition active, effective, self-aware, socially embedded agents, capable of coping interdependently in many respects, and independently in many others, in a wide range of challenging and unchallenging environments. They have a robust form of sociality in terms of attachments to others, concern for, and delight in the well-being of those others for their own sakes, and they have stable, internalized norms of fairness, reciprocity, and reliability. They have initiative, courage, and persistence. Their primal affective responses are differentiated and modulated into emotions proper, and are robustly yoked to their agency and sociality. They have robust abilities to communicate, coordinate, and cooperate with others, and have considerable momentum to do so. They have substantial resistance, resilience, energy, and momentum—both physiologically and psychologically. They are relatively stable—both physiologically and psychologically— with respect to reversals, and their lives have great forwardness (in this case, in the direction of improvement in their abilities and success in their endeavors). They live in an environment in which they have opportunities for the rest, recuperation, and diverting activities necessary for health. They also have opportunities for health-giving forms of pleasure, joy, and elevated or transcendental experience of several sorts—in love, aesthetic experience, contemplative life, religious experience, and in "flow."

Now consider what it takes to get to that kind of health and to sustain it, from the age-adjusted forms of it we might have beginning in infancy, throughout our development to the point at which we can achieve and sustain its adult form, and throughout our decline in old age. And think especially of the environmental dimension of health in this regard. Throughout childhood, adolescence, and young adulthood, human development into fully adult forms of robust health requires appropriate, society-wide allocations of resources. Stability in health at each stage will require stability in social arrangements at each stage. And the introduction of permanent physical or psychological disabilities at any stage in the person's development—or even the probability of such disabilities—will require a social commitment to genuine rehabilitation toward robust health if possible, rather than mere stabilization at a lower level. It will also require societywide accommodations for people for whom rehabilitation by itself cannot fully restore development toward robust health—such as those in the irreversible declines of old age. Furthermore, the development of robust health will require opportunities for each person to experience the pleasures, joys, and elevated or transcendental forms of life that complete and reinforce health.

Given the requirements for habilitation into age-adjusted robust health over an entire life span, for overlapping generations, and given our vulnerability to permanent physical or psychological disabilities, any society with constitutive commitments to the well-being of its citizens will need to sustain social structures that promote its conception of robust health—and thus healthy agency. Pockets of (relative) poverty, or lack of economic resources, education, or supportive social networks, will mean pockets of poor health for the children—poor health that is likely to be sustained and even replicated in the next generation.

Some of this is inevitable and beyond our control. And parts of it that are within our control may best be handled by going after something other than health, strictly construed. The question here is whether the test of success could always be found, ultimately, in the consequences for healthy agency and in scaling the distribution of public resources to such consequences. If so, then habilitation into robustly healthy agency is the appropriate framework and target for distributive justice.

3.2. *Health as a lagging, coarsely discriminating indicator*

It may be objected that the health scale will often not even register rapid or subtle fluctuations in the distribution of goods that might be important for public policy. Thus the health scale might not be an appropriate representative good—or at least the best one. Wealth and income, for example, might go up, down, and up again without showing up at all in consequences for trait-health, and perhaps not even showing up in significant health conditions. Wouldn't this be a disadvantage? Economic resources, it might be urged, are much more finely discriminating. Using wealth and income as the representative good would register rapid fluctuations and small changes.

Or would it? There are lagging economic indicators as well—such as unemployment. And when wealth and income are combined into one scale, we have the same distinction that is found in the health scale: wealth is comparable to a health-trait; income is comparable to a health condition. So wealth and volatile forms of income, combined into one indicator, will not be as finely discriminating as income alone, just as the combination of trait-health and health conditions is not as discriminating as health conditions alone.

And health does have the advantage, again, of being a basic, constitutive good. When fluctuations in other goods do show up in consequences for health, they are clearly matters of concern for any theory of basic justice. The same cannot be said for the reverse. Normative theories differ about whether inequalities of wealth and income, for example, are significant matters of concern as long as they don't have consequences for health.

So at this theory-independent level, health seems the better choice. It is a less prejudicial choice with respect to defining the common ground between normative theories, and it will not be any less sensitive to rapid, subtle fluctuations than the more traditional use of wealth and income.

3.3. *Relevance to distributing a cooperative surplus*

It looks as though the framework proposed here will necessarily be inadequate in the following sense: suppose we organize our cooperative activities and institutions around habilitation into robustly healthy agency for everyone, and we achieve that goal to the extent that is humanly possible. Suppose further that this large-scale, ongoing cooperative effort produces surpluses—either in the form of goods that are of interest to everyone, but not causally related to health, or in the form of goods that are related to health at least indirectly, but which we have in such abundance that we do not need to use them for that purpose. Isn't the distribution of such cooperative surpluses also a matter of basic distributive justice? And wouldn't building such matters into our theory of justice require, by definition, a framework and metric other than habilitation into robustly healthy agency?

The answer is that the framework proposed here has the resources to handle distributive matters above and beyond the target of robustly healthy agency. As a mere metric, rather than a distributive rule, it will not impose a particular rule. But it can be an effective metric for them. For example, it would support a lexically ordered set of priorities such as the following, given in terms of health itself.

The first priority would be to distribute surpluses in a way that does no harm to the level and extent of robustly healthy agency already achieved in society. That will exclude any distribution of surpluses that is damaging to our trait-health *with respect to agency*. Thus it will not exclude distributions that are unanimously chosen, even if those distributions involve some risk for individuals willing to assume them. (We might, for example, assign surpluses to space exploration undertaken by volunteers.) And it will not exclude distributions that are opposed by some people—even vigorously opposed—as long as their consequent unhappiness does not damage their trait-health with respect to agency—as it might do if it made them inconsolably depressed, or resentful.

The second priority would be to distribute surpluses in a way that adds homeostatic stability to what has been achieved and sustains the developmental energy and momentum in such health.

The third priority would be to distribute surpluses in a way that enables members of the society to make progress, consistent with the norms of basic justice, toward lives that exemplify their own favored comprehensive conceptions of the good.

To be consistent with justice under some other distributive rule, the health metric will also suffice as long as healthy agency is causally connected to the goods sought by that rule. That is, I think, sufficient assurance that the habilitation framework and target can handle the general problem of surpluses.

4. Theory All the Way Down: A Public Policy Objection

4.1. *Meta-theoretical prejudices*

There are three parts to the argument of this book: the habilitation framework, the healthy agency target, and the choice of health as the representative good. These three parts appear to be independent in the sense that one could, in principle, accept any one of them while rejecting the other(s). One might accept the argument for framing questions of basic justice in terms of habilitation but reject the idea that we should give special prominence to health and healthy agency. Or one might accept both the habilitation framework and the healthy agency target but reject the choice of health as the representative good. And so on.

The question here is whether this degree of apparent independence among the three parts of the book poses a problem of prejudice: if the part-independence is only apparent rather than real, the apparatus seems to favor similarly unified, top-to-bottom normative theories with interlocking parts. But if the part-independence is real and the parts are genuinely disjunctive, the apparatus seems to favor theories that are similarly loose-jointed.

The three moving parts of this book do look suspiciously unified, from top to bottom, around a closely related set of concepts: habilitation, functional abilities, coping, health, and healthy agency. Further, each subsequent part is developed out of the former ones. All of this suggests that its general structure, even if disjunctive, will match up well with any normative theory that expects to take the very same sorts of arguments all the way to the ground of daily life, keeping the most general principles and methods of the theory intact and adding only rules of thumb, short-cuts, and other techniques as required at different levels of abstraction.

That leaves the question of whether it will match up equally well—in a general, meta-theoretical way—with normative theories that expect to treat matters of justice differently (that is, with somewhat different principles or procedures) at different levels of abstraction.

Consider rule- and motive-utilitarianism. Some utilitarians have apparently expected to apply an uncompromising act-utilitarian principle all the way from the most abstract questions of life and social organization down to the minutia of daily life and public policy about it. But most forms of utilitarianism are much more complex and are self-effacing at various levels: they use uncompromising act-utilitarian reasoning at the highest level of abstraction, but on that basis they also recommend rules of street-level professional conduct (e.g., in obedience to law and law enforcement) that block the detailed application of such calculations, and they recommend the development of motives and dispositions for conduct in daily life (e.g., in friendships and love and daily business transactions) which make utilitarian calculations literally unthinkable in some situations. It looks as though the three parts of this book's theory-independent apparatus might be hostile to making considerations of health unthinkable, or blocking the application of such considerations.

4.2. *Test cases and the presumption against novelty*

The choice of health as the representative good is likely to be the best test case here—especially for people who want to get a workable normative theory of public policy administration about basic justice. For one thing, in that context, given the velocity, complexity, and potential damage of the daily decisions to be made, introducing a novel indexical good may seem deeply dangerous, or at any rate merely academic and ultimately unserious. Better the devils we know: a standard monistic index, such as economic costs and benefits, or a long, pluralistic list of goods, including health, that are not fully commensurable with each other but can be juggled in a perpetual political process of competing interests, aimed at comparative improvements.

The general problems with the devils we know are that all the standard monistic indexes (economic resources, merit, social standing) are simply not plausible as representative goods for many of the things we care about, and the full list of everything we care about in a fundamental way cannot be put on a single scale; that list doesn't seem compatible with an index at all.

I have been arguing that the complete-health-scale is a more comprehensive monistic index than the standard ones, and thus that health is a better choice for the representative good. I will continue that argument in the remainder of the book. But even if it is successful in the abstract, it will not by itself address the question of its adequacy at the level of public policy administration. And it will not address the question of whether, for all its difficulties in resolving the indexing problem, a pluralistic account of representative goods might not still be better than the choice of health as *the* representative good.

It will be helpful here to consider a test case in some detail—one directed to matters of public policy and one that doesn't merely wave away the indexing problem but rather proposes a practical way around it.

4.3. *A particularly strong test case: Plural disadvantages*

In *Disadvantage* (2007), Jonathan Wolff and Avner de-Shalit, working within a generally utilitarian public policy framework and an egalitarian, interventionist, welfare state context, make a striking public policy proposal about what such governments should do to deal with unevenly distributed disadvantages.

Wolff and de-Shalit, following Sen and Nussbaum's fundamental insight, interpret persistent social disadvantages as deficits in the capabilities and functionings crucial for well-being in one's environment. And they, like Sen and Nussbaum, regard such capabilities as irreducibly plural. For public policy reasons, however, Wolff and de-Shalit want to focus almost entirely on functionings, since they are more directly available for measurement than the underlying traits or capabilities. They begin with Nussbaum's list of central capabilities, together with some additional items they think might plausibly be included. They then submit the list to a reality check (against the suspicion that it might be too intellectualized and culture bound for public policy purposes) by explaining it to a range of social service professionals in societies of particular interest, and then interviewing them at length about what might be missing from the list, or what should be deleted from it.

There is a great deal in Wolff and de-Shalit's project that is either supportive of or challenging for the habilitation framework. A supportive element is their finding, both from philosophical and empirical sources, that reflective people engaged in the provision of social services cite people's fundamental need for *secure* functionings as a central concern for basic justice. The analog to the concept of health described in Chapters 4–5 is in its emphasis on functional abilities that are reliable, stable, and strong in a given environment.

A challenging element is that Wolff and de-Shalit argue against the notion that there can be a single scale along which all disadvantages can be ranked and compared so as to identify the worst-off members of society, the next worst-off, and so forth. That is, they do not think that the so-called indexing problem can be solved in that way. Rather, they propose a method for working around it.

The survey of practitioners. Consider first the interviews—mostly of social workers and other practitioners—as reported in *Disadvantage* (Ch. 2). Wolff and de-Shalit's interview process, which initially covered about 100 respondents, was extensive, and interviewers discussed with each respondent, item by item, an amended version of Nussbaum's list of central capabilities. They report that some of their interviewees objected to item 1 (life) on Nussbaum's list, saying it was a precondition at best, not a separate element of a good life. In responses to various other items, as well as to item 2 (bodily health), there was comment on the importance of mental health as well as bodily health—a matter, incidentally, that the habilitation framework tackles directly, and prominently. Some people thought there was too much packed into Nussbaum's item 4 (sense, imagination, and thought), and that item 6 (practical reason) was strange. Item 8 (other species) was not widely approved by the respondents, though item 9 (play) was. Item 10 (control of one's environment) got approval except from some who objected to its mention of property rights. But in general, though there was much disagreement about matters of emphasis and about what was left out of Nussbaum's list, Wolff and de-Shalit think it held up well.

For the purposes of their interviews, the authors added an item of a libertarian sort, quite distinct from anything on Nussbaum's list, partly to see whether the interviewees were just "nodding along" rather than thinking carefully about the categories, and partly to see whether there was a general sympathy for the idea of complete independence as a goal for an optimal human life (51). This was vigorously rejected by a small group, vigorously endorsed by a small group, and vigorously reinterpreted by the rest.

For other reasons, the authors added three other items to Nussbaum's list, in the categories of doing good to others, living in a law-abiding fashion, and understanding the law (50–51). The first of these (doing good to others) was enthusiastically endorsed by almost all the interviewees. It is of course implicit in parts of Nussbaum's list, but the emphasis on benevolence, caring, and gratitude in this separate item were gratifying to most interviewees. It is notable that a substantial number of interviewees understood gratitude in terms of reciprocity.

The second of these items (the ability to live in a law-abiding fashion) caused some controversy among those who thought that breaking the law, or cheating, was either not so bad (the rich do it) or was sometimes the right thing to do. The authors insist on its importance, however, and think it was misunderstood. What they have in mind is people who want very much to live within the law but find themselves without that option—at least without it in the sense that for survival, they have to do some things that are illegal.

The third of these additions (the ability to understand the law) got general agreement, but crystallized something for many interviewees which came out when they were asked whether they wanted to add anything to the list of fourteen items that had been presented to them. A widespread consensus emerged that somewhat surprised the authors. Many interviewees suggested that the ability to communicate verbally was a fundamentally important aspect of functioning and needed to be made explicit in the list (60). Since most of the interviewees were social service professionals who work in areas where many immigrants do not speak the local language in a way that makes them independent of translators, this item makes sense. And it is interesting that while language ability fits naturally into the capabilities approach, it needs to be brought to our attention in a special way, to ensure that it gets the appropriate amount of attention in normative theory. (Health, as robustly healthy agency in a given environment, is fully compatible with that.)

Relation to the use of health as the representative good. Wolff and de-Shalit might accept as useful or at any rate harmless the first part of the argument here—the habilitation framework. And they might accept the centrality of complete health and healthy agency to many of the functionings (capabilities) that are central to basic justice. But the healthy agency target and the choice of health as a representative good appear to be incompatible with their primary public policy proposal, and it may appear that the whole structure of the habilitation framework is (inadvertently) set up to be prejudicial to their proposal.

This is not the case, however, for the following reasons.

The indexing problem. Wolff and de-Shalit take the indexing problem very seriously and do not think it can be ignored by focusing on matters of comparative justice (Sen) or be avoided by setting mandatory thresholds for each item on the list (Nussbaum). They think the impossibility of a monistic solution to the indexing problem for all central functionings taken together can be established on formal, meta-theoretical grounds (24–35, 89). But they go on to propose a work-around solution to the indexing problem that leaves the plurality of goods intact while allowing us to identify the very worst-off members of society, and to move forward step by step toward rectifying disadvantage (Chs. 5–7).

The workaround solution they offer turns out to be a particularly good test case. They drop the whole idea of using any particular functioning as a representative good. Instead, they suggest constructing what they call functioning maps for representative individuals—maps that chart the levels and relationships of all the central functionings (capabilities). It is then those maps that are compared with each other to find the worst-off members of society. They proceed roughly as follows.

First, they concede that there are useful ways of solving indexing problems for subsets of seemingly disparate functionings. Indeed, they "take for granted that it is possible to measure the functioning level of each representative individual for each functioning" (89). Further, they acknowledge that a given functioning (as we might identify it for practical purposes) may be quite complex and decomposable into separate functions with separate scales. Their example is decathlon scoring, and their discussion of it makes clear that their objection to a global monistic solution to the indexing problem—one that puts all the central functionings on the same scale—does not cut against the possibility of constructing a complete-health-scale of the sort proposed here (99–100).

Second, they argue that the indexing problem cannot be handled by dividing the government into sectors (education, health, housing, transportation, and so forth), developing an index for each and proceeding to apply distributive principles. For one thing, that doesn't solve the prior questions about how much of the budget to allocate to each sector. For another, it doesn't fully recognize the ways in which a problem or its rectification in one sector creates a problem in another (89–92). Further, they note that adopting a threshold requirement for each sector or functioning within it does not solve these problems, since it doesn't give us a way of making allocations when resources are scarce—at least, not without assigning weights to these things, which will either be arbitrary or depend on an implicit overall solution to the indexing problem after all (92–94).

Third, they emphasize that while their list of central functionings is ultimately plural, empirical investigation shows that it contains six "high weight" items, generally agreed by interviewees to be the most important, and that functioning levels generally agreed to be especially salient typically show themselves in clusters that cross these high weight categories (104–6). Moreover, they cite empirical evidence to the effect that there may be a "convergence" between perceived disadvantages and perceived bad health, together with various psychological and social factors (122–25).

Fourth, Wolff and de-Shalit emphasize the ways in which clusters of disadvantages and advantages are often *dynamic*—causally connected, as in feedback loops and spirals: insecurity in economic resources begets poverty, which begets compromises in nutrition and living conditions, which beget poor health, which begets a decline in the ability to work, which begets additional economic insecurity . . . and so on, downward. Some of those clusters are especially *corrosive*, either because they become increasingly encompassing (bringing more and more functionings into the cluster) or because they become increasingly self-perpetuating. Others are especially fertile in their ability to overcome disadvantages (120–22).

Fifth, the authors emphasize throughout the book that for public policy and justice, what matters is not simply some given range and level of functioning but rather the *security* (stability, reliability) of such functioning (65–72).

Sixth, when they come to make a general recommendation for public policy, Wolff and de-Shalit suggest that what the government should do is to *de-cluster* disadvantages, beginning with the most corrosive clusters, in ways that reestablish not only a defensible level of functioning for each element involved but make that functioning secure (Chs. 8–10). (Advantages cluster also, of course, and some of those clusters are especially self-reinforcing, and thus self-securing. Ultimately, one wants to replace corrosive clusters of disadvantages with fertile, self-securing clusters of advantages.)

4.4. *Lack of prejudice toward this test case*

Let us assume that Wolff and de-Shalit's normative policy recommendation is sound. Then that part of their normative theory will be compatible with the choice of health as the representative good if and only if (1) it is plausible to think that complete health is necessarily involved, either directly or indirectly, in all corrosive clusters of disadvantages and self-securing clusters of advantages, and (2) health tracks (dis)advantage closely enough, and with enough sensitivity, to be a good index to it.

If those conditions can be met, then presumably any normative approach to public policy will have to recognize this in *some* way. Whether this is done by explicitly choosing health as the representative good or whether (as in Wolff and de-Shalit's project) it is done by recognizing the role health plays in a "pragmatic" approach to public policy that operates without explicit reference to any single representative good is not a crucial issue. One should be able to build a top-to-bottom normative theory or a loose-jointed one within this theory-independent framework.

Implicitly, the argument for the habilitation framework is that complete health (in the region of robustly healthy agency) meets those two conditions. The form of the argument on this matter is applicable not only to this test case but to the general problem of normative theories that want to proceed without the choice of health as the representative good.

Complete health, and in particular healthy agency, is always a necessary part of achieving *secure* functionings of all the central sorts. Equipping people with food, housing, work, income, wealth, education, and goods other than health will not yield secure functionings for such people if they lack secure healthy-agency functioning. Think of wealthy, well-educated people in favorable social environments whose lives are repeatedly disrupted and restored by persistent cycles of alcohol or drug abuse, or persistent disabling levels of anxiety. They lack secure functionings even if a welfare state guarantees unending (but only intermittently effective) rehabilitation.

Moreover, healthy agency is a sensitive index that tracks (dis)advantage closely, both in terms of risk and actual damage. A risk to healthy agency always compromises the *security* of other functionings, since it is necessary for them, as noted above. And a risk to healthy agency constitutes an outright risk for all the centrally important functionings: without substantial positive health, human beings do not thrive over the long-term; if they do not thrive, their health wanes or withers; if their health wanes or withers, everything else is put at risk. So health is a sensitive index to risk.

It is also a sensitive index to actual damage. The level of damage (or risk of damage) to healthy agency that is associated with damage to other central functionings tracks to a remarkable extent our judgments about whether the latter are properly matters of concern for basic justice. (See Chapter 9 for further argument on this point.)

None of this means, of course, that health is the only sort of functioning we care about. Nor does it mean that the most effective methods for de-clustering disadvantages (or re-clustering advantages) will always be directly aimed at improving health. It simply means that our success in dealing with disadvantages will always depend on our success in making the relevant improvements in health—either because those improvements are necessary to improving all the other functionings involved or are necessary to improving the *security* of those functionings.

Part 3

Healthy Agency and the Norms of Basic Justice

Preface to Part Three

In all hospitable and potentially hospitable environments, people face at least three distinct habilitative tasks: (1) getting the habilitation sufficient for their own welfare, through their own efforts and the efforts of others; (2) helping to habilitate others to the extent necessary; and (3) helping to habilitate the physical and social environment where necessary—for example, by making efforts to transform a merely survivable or minimally hospitable environment into a genuinely hospitable one.

The extent to which agents understand these tasks and how they might be accomplished depends on the extent to which the agents are self-aware, knowledgeable about habilitative possibilities and necessities, and capable of practical reasoning. The extent to which agents actually engage in those tasks and the ways in which they limit their efforts depends on the nature of their motivation and abilities as agents.

Chapter 7 shows how the functional abilities and motivation of basically healthy agents are concerned with the subject matter of justice. Chapter 8 shows how those elements of basically healthy agency run parallel to, and can be represented as, norms of basic justice. Agentic health motivates many of the norms of basic justice, is consistent with others, and puts persistent pressure on them to narrow, refine, and extend the consensus they represent—not in the direction of a particular theory of justice but in the direction of an equal distribution throughout the population of the things necessary for basic health.

7

Healthy Agency and Its
Behavioral Tendencies

This chapter and the next are extrapolations from the compressed account of the circumstances of habilitation given in Chapter 2, and the accounts of health and agency given in Chapters 3–6.

1. Dispositions toward Health and Habilitation

Heterogeneous motivation. Any reasonably full account of the circumstances of habilitation will describe a heterogeneous and potentially conflicting and even incoherent collection of motivational elements characteristic of human persons and their behavioral tendencies: egocentrism versus sociality; mutual advantage versus mutual aid; acquisitiveness, possessiveness, greed and envy versus beneficence, generosity, cooperative labor, and admiration of others' achievements. Unless these and many other motivational elements are coherently organized and modulated with respect to each other, the resulting chaos of impulsiveness, ambivalence, and motivational conflict makes reliably competent functioning impossible. And unless the form of coherent organization and modulation is also strategically sound with respect to interaction with the physical and social environment, reliably competent functioning will also be impossible.

Consider the following very partial list: human beings have strongly motivated first-order physiological and psychological drives for survival (air, water, thermoregulation, food, shelter, clothing), as well as for habilitative social relationships—especially those related to the satisfaction of survival needs and primal physiological appetites. We also have strongly motivated first-order psychological needs for security with respect to survival and habilitative social relationships; for the acquisition of resources and the security of such resources; for attachment and security in the benefits of such attachments; and for gratification of appetites beyond those needed for survival and habilitative social relationships.

Then second-order drives are generated by the way in which the first-order drives have been satisfied, or not, as the case may be. These include strongly motivated efforts to improve the effectiveness of the agency powers necessary for pursuing the satisfaction of first-order drives. Thus we are motivated to monitor such needs (locating their sources, identifying methods of satisfying them, assessing the opportunities for satisfying them, identifying methods for taking those opportunities, assessing the strategic factors in the pursuit of those methods and opportunities, assessing the consistency of such pursuits with respect to other needs and goals), and we are motivated to find a competent balance of decisiveness, resoluteness, and persistence in the pursuit of such goals as well as to adapt all of this to changed circumstances as we proceed.

In addition, we have third-order drives generated by the way in which the second-order ones have been satisfied, or not. These include achieving a stable, coherent, well-organized structure for these heterogeneous drives—what amounts to a harmonization of them, expressed in stable, homeostatic physiological and psychological traits that are nonetheless labile enough to adapt to predictable changes in the physical and social environment.

Good basic health yields a coherent motivational structure, and the pursuit of such health is thereafter strongly motivated. For human beings, the reliably competent functioning involved in good basic health includes a coherent, self-regulating structure of physiological traits necessary for survival and the development of the organism. And it includes a similar structure of psychological traits—one that functions competently, and reliably so, with heterogeneous motivational material. So to say that the heterogeneity of our motivational endowments and personalities creates a strongly motivated drive toward a coherent, self-sustaining motivational structure (and away from an incoherent or self-defeating one) is to say that we have a strongly motivated drive toward basic eudaimonistic good health.

Diversity of coherent, self-sustaining motivational structures. It is hard to imagine any genuinely hospitable environment in which there will not be significant diversity in basically healthy personalities. There is bound to be a large array of at least subtly distinct combinations of personal traits and motivational structures that will lie in the region between excess and deficiency—that is, in the region of reliably competent functioning—in any given hospitable environment. Some people will be taciturn, solitary, and emotionally remote. Others will be talkative, gregarious, and emotionally accessible. Some will be guarded, apprehensive, and reluctant to cooperate except in projects guaranteed to prevent bad things from happening. Others will be unguarded, adventurous, and eager to cooperate in risky projects that might make good things happen. Some will be backward looking, others forward-looking—and so forth, on and on.

One can imagine genuinely hospitable environments in which options for thriving are very limited, so that (compared to other environments) the range of reliably competent personality traits is very narrow in absolute terms. Life in antiquity on a remote, sparsely populated frontier might be an example, if we imagine there is a small number of essential tasks and a barely adequate labor supply for each. Presumably, human beings would generally be motivated to enlarge those options, or at least to habilitate themselves to function competently elsewhere, if necessary. Nonetheless, for present purposes it is important to note that even the most restrictive hospitable environment in absolute terms will have much the same kind of diversity in relative terms. The differences between people will still look large relative to each other, even though they may look very small against those in less restrictive environments. People will still have to deal with others who seem dramatically different from themselves, but who are not pathological, and they will have to deal with others who are dangerously excessive or deficient, perhaps to a pathological degree, and perhaps not. The types of habilitative problems are the same no matter how restrictive or nonrestrictive the hospitable environment may be.

Several clusters of these habilitative problems are particularly salient here. They concern the presence or absence of psychological traits necessary for creating or sustaining a hospitable environment. This inevitably requires the ability to cope with collective action problems: achieving the necessary degree of interpersonal coordination and cooperation; resolving interpersonal conflicts; dealing with external threats to social survival; dealing with internal threats from secessionists, conscientious disobedience, free riders, grifters, violent criminals, and so forth. We will get to such matters in Section 2.2 of this chapter.

Vulnerability to ill health. Another of the circumstances of habilitation, of course, is our persistent vulnerability to ill health. This has four closely interrelated sources. One is the fact that our individual endowments or developed capabilities are never strong enough to immunize us completely from physical or psychological disease, injury, deficit, disability, or distress. Another is that inhospitable environments promote such ill health, in ways that even the best habilitative efforts cannot overcome. (Think of landscapes in which malaria is endemic.) A third is that we are vulnerable to each other in this respect—not only because we injure each other through accidents, violence, or abuse but also because we are vectors of infectious disease.[1] And the fourth is that individual ill health and inhospitable environments can become self-perpetuating—as, for example, when one aspect of the psychological ill health involved is a set of intense, self-defeating attachments to preserving the status quo. (Think of social environments in which a caste system is deeply institutionalized, and the consequent differentials in life expectancy and quality of life are accepted by all, as somehow deserved.)

---

[1] See Battin, Francis, Jacobson, and Smith, *The Patient as Victim and Vector* (2009).

Self-perpetuating forms of physical and psychological ill health are pervasive in human political history. They produce carefully habilitated psychological blindness to the ruthlessness, cruelty, violence, domination, and systematic subordination or enslavement of some for the advancement of others, together with carefully habilitated behaviors of similar blindness and submission in those who are subordinated or enslaved.[2]

Some of these practices may well have gotten started as rational choices by everyone involved. In a barely survivable physical environment, people may not be able to avoid such temporary arrangements and thus subject themselves to a method for conscripting people for certain tasks, or risks, or even self-sacrifice. Some lifeboat cases, in which a self-appointed leader enlists a crew, assigns tasks, and limits or reduces the number of passengers, are examples. But it is unfortunately not difficult to see the many routes through which such practices become self-perpetuating on a grand scale.[3]

Habilitation toward genuinely hospitable environments and away from those that perpetuate ill health is strongly motivated. Nonetheless, as long as habilitation toward basic health is strongly motivated, and as long as agents who are so motivated are able to recognize forms of ill health perpetuated by their physical and social environments, they will also be motivated to habilitate such environments. It follows that the habilitation of survivable environments into genuinely habilitative ones (those in which succeeding generations of some human beings living in communities regularly survive in good health, for long periods, with time and energy to spend on more than survival activities) is also strongly motivated.

2. Dispositions about the Subject Matter of Justice

Strongly motivated as they may be toward basic good health, including complex rational agency, and toward making the necessary habilitative efforts for those things, individual human beings acting alone are not able to achieve and sustain

---

[2] For an analysis of slavery that makes especially vivid its psychological impact on both slave and slaveholder, see part one of Orlando Patterson, *Slavery and Social Death: A Comparative Study* (1992). It is clear from his analysis that in some especially hostile environments, we should be hesitant about concluding that the psychological consequences, or causes, of slavery are necessarily indicative of psychological ill health. But of course the absence of ill health is not the whole issue here. We want to know also whether basic good health is consistent with sorts of capabilities and motivational dispositions involved in creating and sustaining the institution of slavery. If Patterson is right to say that turning slavery into a self-perpetuating institution has always involved a deliberately, elaborately, and ritualistically imposed form of "social death" on the slave, then it is hard to think that any such institution could be consistent with the aspects of basic good psychological health described in Section 2.

[3] *United States v. Holmes* 26 F.Cas. 360 (1842) is one such lifeboat case. But for an example on a grand scale lasting millennia, see Toby Wilkinson, *The Rise and Fall of Ancient Egypt* (2011).

them. They need help from each other—specifically, help of a habilitative sort. And such mutual assistance must be multigenerational to succeed.

Reliably competent functioning (good basic health) will therefore include the motivational elements and coping abilities that make mutual assistance possible, and possible to sustain, in a multigenerational way. From the point of view of an individual agent, some of this assistance will address the individual's own welfare. Some of it will address others' welfare. And still more will address what is needed to create and sustain a genuinely hospitable environment.

For expository convenience, both with respect to previous parts of the discussion and to Chapter 8, I will organize the discussion in terms of these clusters of related traits: sociality, individuality, cooperation, and regulation. Each of these clusters represents a set of habilitative problems that human beings face throughout their lives—including habilitation and rehabilitation into basic health. For example, much of the habilitation we need is provided for us through our physical and social environments. As a consequence, the motivational and behavioral traits of basic health must include the sort of functioning required to prompt, accept, and use the habilitation provided—as well as to maintain or improve the environments themselves. But much of the necessary habilitation must also be self-provided, and thus the motivational and behavioral traits of basic health must include the sort of functioning required to develop and sustain agency that is competent to provide such self-habilitation. Individual agents must become autonomous to the extent that they can monitor social interactions so as to avoid the ones that are self-defeating—either by being harmful to basic health generally, or to agency itself. The following clusters of traits stand out as especially important in these respects.

2.1. *Sociality*

The social environments within which habilitation of all sorts typically occurs are characterized by a variety of interactive social relationships. Basic health—competent functioning in such relationships—is thus characterized by certain important forms of mutuality. Many of the forms of mutuality mentioned below are familiar as normative principles with the same names, derived philosophically from prior metaphysical or moral principles or analyses of moral reasoning.[4] The

---

[4] Recognition, for example, mutual or not, often appears in accounts of human psychological or political life indebted to Hegel's speculative metaphysical psychology—especially in his accounts of the emergence of self-consciousness, his analysis of the master/slave relationship, and the development of an objective concept of rightness and rights. As used here, however, mutual recognition, along with mutual respect, has a more modest function, more like the one that appears in some contemporary normative moral theories (e.g., in Scanlon, 1998). Nonetheless, the philosophical importance of recognition is by some accounts very broad and deep. See Schmidt and Zurn, *The Philosophy of Recognition: Historical and Contemporary Perspectives* (2010), especially pp. 1–20.

accounts given here are meant to move in the other direction: from descriptions of human motivation within the framework of actual habilitative concerns toward normative principles that might be generated from them.

Mutual recognition. One crucial form of mutuality central to basic health is the mutual recognition of others as other individuals and interest in them as such. One way in which this begins for infants is with intense interest in human faces (and comparable interest among older children and adults in watching infant faces for signs of recognition). This early fascination on both sides then typically develops into increasingly complex forms of attentiveness and responsiveness each to the other. Attentive watching and listening on the part of infants soon develops into responses designed to elicit repetition of some things and cessation of other things—and is predicated on prelinguistic forms of memory and anticipation. But the habilitative success of such behavior on the part of the infant depends on getting similarly attentive watching, listening, and ultimately appropriate responses from others. The signaling involved in such responses then typically develops toward more elaborate forms of communication, predicated ultimately on fluency in the use of language, and highly articulated representations of the self, others, and the physical and social environment. Again however, this is dependent on appropriate communicative responses from others.

A parallel path of recognition and response involves an infant's efforts to mirror the things others do (in terms of facial expression, attentiveness, vocalization, gestures, and so forth), which then typically develop into deliberate imitation and ultimately into increasingly complex, continually surprising, mutually delighting responses. (An example frequently noted by parents is a child's developing capability to engage in genuine conversation even prior to much language acquisition.)

Mutual respect and honor. Mutual recognition can occur in disrespectful ways as well as respectful ones. For human beings, the respectful kinds seem especially necessary for habilitation into basic health. These are the kinds of recognition which honor what Rawls calls the separateness of persons, and which honor every habilitative effort toward good basic health and the hospitable social environments required by it. Adults with robustly healthy forms of agency differ considerably in the extent to which they are dependent on specific rewards for specific conduct. So, apparently, do children. But the psychological importance of reinforcement is well known, and the presence or absence of it in the form of general acknowledgment of one's worthiness of respect is also well known. Without it, the social environment is not genuinely hospitable, and good basic health is probably not even achievable. Furthermore, when it is achieved, if all mutual respect is removed, basic good health is eventually eroded.

Mutual respect for personal boundaries, necessities for identity, and personal holdings. Just as mutual recognition leads to mutual respect and honor, mutual respect leads to an appreciation of the personal boundaries of others and of what they believe belongs to them personally. This appreciation of personal boundaries, identities, and holdings has a source in self-respect as well (see Individuality later in the chapter), and is extended by analogy to others. But it also has an independent motivation by way of mutuality and is reflected back to one's own case to reinforce that aspect of self-respect. These notions of boundaries, boundary keeping, and the necessary goods of agency and identity are important circumstances of habilitation, which often conflict with other important behavioral dispositions. Reliably competent functioning in a social environment requires a coherent form of agency that reconciles such conflicts. Mutual respect (along with other things) helps to achieve that and is thus an element of basic psychological health.

Mutual (radiating) benevolence and solidarity. Mutual benevolence also arises from mutual recognition and mutual respect. Since these forms of mutuality have their earliest, most profound, and most consistent development in intimate relationships, and continue to have their most immediate importance there and in other personal relationships, mutual benevolence tends to arise first as radiating benevolence. That is, it tends to be the most powerful nearest the core of those fundamental, intimate relationships, growing progressively weaker as the relationships are more remote.

Such widely shared dispositions toward mutual benevolence amount to a form of solidarity that has a similar radiating structure. One's own psychological well-being is causally linked to the well-being of others—most strongly to the well-being of one's intimates and most weakly to the well-being of those farthest away—either in physical, social, or psychological terms.

As the world effectively becomes closer—through easier travel, more vivid and immediate forms of communication, more general social and commercial networks and so forth—radiating benevolence and solidarity may begin to approximate something resembling the impartial, universal benevolence recommended by some normative theories of justice. But there does not seem to be a source for such universal benevolence in basic good health itself, and I suspect it is only an unstable resemblance to it that we sometimes experience through travel, correspondence, narrative art, and television coverage of human suffering in war, famine, and natural disasters. Perhaps there is such a source in perfect health.

It is clear, however, that insofar as mutual recognition and mutual respect are stable elements of basic health, so too are mutual radiating benevolence and the forms of solidarity it generates.

Mutual (radiating) beneficence. Insofar as a social relationship is marked by mutual benevolence and solidarity, beneficence is also motivated, as the translation of benevolent motives into beneficial conduct. The extent of the beneficence varies in obvious ways, along with the strength of the benevolence and solidarity under-lying it, the need for it, and the way conflicting circumstances of habilitation are resolved. Some of these matters are revisited in the discussion of reciprocity and related matters further in the chapter. Some of these provide independent sources for beneficence, and some of them tend to limit such conduct. Considering the forms of reliably competent agency that might be found in hospitable environ-ments generally, it seems necessary to conclude that the beneficence characteristic of basic good health would also be multisourced and limited.

Conviviality. In a social environment marked by mutuality of all these sorts (recognition, respect, radiating benevolence and solidarity, beneficence), soci-ality typically develops some momentum toward conviviality—seeking and enjoying the company of others for its own sake, along with playfulness and good humor for the sake of others. It is unclear how much of this is a constituent of basic good health—that is, merely reliably competent functioning in a hospi-table environment—when it is traced only to these forms of mutuality. But con-viviality also has motivational sources in collective rituals, celebrations, public entertainments and performances, and in patterns of hospitality. To the extent that those things are necessary for getting widespread social cooperation, for example, conviviality has another connection to habilitative tasks, and thus to reliably competent functioning.

2.2. *Individuality*

The discussion turns away now from forms of mutuality to elements of individuality— self-regarding traits found in basic good health that are both necessary elements of reliably competent functioning in a given environment and at the same time give significant shape to it.

The discussion of eudaimonistic health in earlier chapters, together with an appreciation of the circumstances of habilitation, make it clear that a great many things can in principle fall under this heading of individuality. But for present purposes, I will concentrate on a cluster of traits with special significance for the self-habilitative aspects of life. That means an immediate focus on some self-habilitative traits that are necessary for integrated, competent agency—the sort of agency that can cope with the heterogeneous nature of human motivation, and the novelty of the challenges this presents throughout life. But this discussion will also focus on the self-preserving and self-habilitative demands of social life in at least minimally hospitable physical and social environments.

The argument throughout assumes that basic good health is strongly motivated away from self-destructive and self-defeating activity, and toward self-protective and self-realizing activity. This is not at all inconsistent with the notion that the self is the product of development in a social environment in which the individual's initial endowments and behavioral tendencies are shaped and sometimes transformed. Individuality is indeed a social product, beginning with sexual reproduction and proceeding through the habilitative efforts of others in a given physical and social environment. But human individuals in good health are not social insects. Human agency of every type, from purely animal agency onward, exhibits important forms of separateness from others and from activities whose only end is the organic perfection of the human social organism. So one characteristic form of human agency is agentic individuality—goals for oneself that serve oneself, if necessary against others, and against physical and social systems.

In that context, the following aspects of individuality stand out as especially important features of basic good health. They are familiar and uncontroversial. The aim of the argument here will be merely to organize the account of them so as to make it blindingly obvious that the conception of basic good health used here entails that (1) people in such good health have some dispositions of all the sorts described, though they may vary significantly in how, and how well, they operate in a given environment; (2) and that those dispositions are about matters central to basic justice.

Self-knowledge. Considerable self-knowledge is obviously necessary for self-habilitation toward a complex, difficult to achieve end. Basic good health, and especially the form of competent agency it requires, is such an end. But getting the kind of self-knowledge required for reliably competent functioning in a given environment—that is, the kind required for basic good health—is an ongoing difficulty. The environment is constantly changing, often subtly. We are opaque to ourselves in various ways, sometimes deliberately, through refusal or avoidance of self-examination. When we engage in self-examination, we often construct an account of our histories and possibilities that is mistaken, again sometimes deliberately, through attempts to present ourselves in a way that serves purposes other than self-knowledge. And of course our motivations are heterogeneous and conflicting, and they often arise in surprising ways from unconscious sources. All of this makes the task of acquiring self-knowledge—crucial as it is for competent functioning— a fundamental and continuing activity of basically healthy human agents.

Practical wisdom. Translating self-knowledge into effective self-habilitation toward basic good health obviously requires practical wisdom—the sort of practical intelligence required for putting self-knowledge to work in achieving and sustaining reliably competent agentic functioning. The standard forms of outcome-oriented practical reasoning are obviously a large part of this: means-end calculations designed to find possible paths to a given outcome and to evaluate the probability of success for those possibilities, as well as the risks and benefits.

But in strategic situations, such as those in which outcomes depend upon the reactions of others to what we do as much as they depend on our own actions, we have to have the sort of practical intelligence needed to choose the right strategy. In many cases the initial outcome we had in mind will change as we proceed in terms of the strategy we choose.

We need practical intelligence in two forms of strategic reasoning. One is inward looking, so as to anticipate and deal with our own responses to decisions we might make. The classic cases of ambivalence, weakness of will, and resistance of other sorts make it evident that we often have to choose a strategy (rather than an outcome) to deal with inner conflicts. ("I thought this was going to be easy. I want to do it. I constantly, passionately want to do it. But every time I try, I find myself so conflicted and depressed I can't even get started.") The other sort of strategic reasoning is outward looking, so as to anticipate and deal with responses that might come from other individuals or from impersonal sources in the physical or social environment.

Here again there are standard forms of practical reasoning involved, in addition to the purely outcome-oriented kinds. All of these things, however, depend on finding non-self-destructive and non-self-defeating solutions—or failing that, a modus vivendi that allows us to postpone the solution. Sometimes these things can be managed by sequencing: not eliminating one side of the conflict or the other but rather satisfying both, in a sequence that resolves the conflict. When that is not possible, there will sometimes be an evident solution in terms of priorities. When setting priorities fails, there may be forms of accommodation or adjustment that are non-self-destructive and non-self-defeating.

These are obvious methods, but their wise practical applications depend on two things (other than self-knowledge and skillful practical reasoning). One is a vivid appreciation of the range of possibilities that are damaging but actually non-self-destructive and non-self-defeating for a given individual in a given environment. Basic good health is robust, and part of its robustness is its homeostatic stability and resilience. For most conflicts, either internal ones or interpersonal ones, there are some sorts of losses that are tolerable because genuinely substitutable benefits can be found. For other losses, for which no substitutable benefits are possible, genuinely compensatory benefits can be found. And for losses without the possibility of either substitutable or compensatory benefits, resilience and rehabilitative measures may maintain basic good health. Leaving aside questions of equal treatment for the moment, no-win situations may sometimes be decided in favor of those who are least resilient to the losses involved. (Think of the deep pockets rationale for decisions in some tort cases.) And if both sides of the conflict are resilient, and equally so, a coin toss may do.

The other element of practical wisdom in these situations, however, is a vivid appreciation of the limits of resilience: the points at which the losses at stake are genuinely incompatible with continued basic good health, or rehabilitation into it.

When that is true, and the choice is forced, the options available are obviously limited; irreversible damage of some sort is inevitable. Even so, practical wisdom can sometimes find solutions in other factors. The first step in finding such solutions, however, is finding the limits of resilience.

Impossibilities and necessities. The things that are necessary for habilitation into basic good health, like the things that make it impossible, are ultimately matters of fact. But insofar as even simple rational agency and autonomy are involved in our activity, beliefs about those facts, true or false, implicit or explicit, directly determine matters of motivation and behavior with respect to them.

When an individual comes to have a *fixed* belief about the impossibilities and necessities for habilitation in his or her own case, the motivational and behavioral consequences are potent, stark, dichotomous, and either impulsive or adamant. Impossibilities are translated into thoughts about boundaries, limits, and demands of a negative sort. "I cannot survive this in good health" becomes "I cannot tolerate this" or "I must not be expected to endure this" or "I will not be subjected to it." Behavioral consequences range from rebellion or other nonnegotiable forms of resistance to nonnegotiable forms of acquiescence and resignation. Necessities, by contrast, are translated into necessary goods and demands of a positive sort: "I cannot survive in good health without this" becomes "I must not be denied it" or "I must have it." The behavioral consequences are similarly wide ranging but also nonnegotiable.

Practical wisdom, as a part of basic good health, involves a prudent appreciation of both the advantages and disadvantages of such fixed beliefs. On the one hand, the motivation they provide can be advantageous even when they turn out to be false: we may pursue habilitative benefits and resist habilitative damage more zealously than we pursue mere possibilities. Sometimes that zealousness turns out to have habilitative benefits. On the other hand, the same zealousness can sometimes make matters worse by foreclosing habilitative possibilities one has mistakenly ignored. This can happen either when the zealousness takes the form of fighting as if to the death over something that is not in fact lethal, or resigning oneself to death when conditions are in fact survivable.

Practical wisdom in these matters also involves a prudent appreciation of the difficulty of identifying impossibilities and necessities accurately, in individual cases. There are many clear cases: flat-out nonsurvivable environments, for example, or nonsurvivable courses of action. But basic good health is by definition reliably competent functioning in a given environment or range of environments. And an important part of its reliability is its adaptability and resilience. So the range of genuine habilitative possibilities between the poles of impossibility and necessity is likely to be large once basic good health has been achieved. And a single counterexample will defeat any claim of habilitative impossibility or necessity at any point toward or within basic good health. The claim will be defeated by the existence of a single navigable and accessible path toward achieving or sustaining good health. Hospitable, and potentially hospitable environments have many such paths; that is what makes them hospitable. Human beings in basic good health can usually find and navigate at least one of them.

Nonetheless, the ways in which these possibilities and necessities for habilitation differ from individual to individual in a given environment are bewilderingly complex. Some of the differences are attributable to idiosyncratic individual endowments. Some are attributable to the extent and nature of the individual's history of habilitation, or to the extent of the idiosyncratic range of environments in which the individual can remain in good health, or to the particular way in which the heterogeneous elements of health (especially the motivational structure of healthy agency) have been made reliably coherent and competent to cope.

The subtleties of the functioning involved in any given individual are often opaque, both to the individual involved and to others, and cannot even be determined after the fact. ("You are certainly much stronger now. But I am no closer to understanding exactly why that happened in your case, and fails in so many others.") Consequently, explanations and predictions about the limits of habilitation and resilience in particular cases are often elusive, if not downright baffling. The best we seem able to do in the subtle cases is to construct revisable probability distributions for large populations and expect to find many inexplicable exceptions.

All of this is so commonsensical that it seems unproblematic to conclude that prudence in all these respects will be included in the form of practical wisdom characteristic of basic good health—or rather, characteristic of the forms of basically healthy rational agency. Like every other element of motivational structure and behavioral tendencies individuals, however, the extent and nature of such prudence will be quite varied.

Self-command, courage, persistence, assessment, and revision. A necessary step in applying practical wisdom to decision making and conduct, of course, is what is often called self-command. Most broadly speaking, this is the agentic ability to transform values into evaluative priorities, priorities into goals, goals into a set of available options, deliberation about the options into plans about which options to pursue and how to proceed. Then all of that must be transformed into choices, decisions, and ultimately actions. Along the way, problems of self-defeating incoherence, ambivalence, motivation, and inanition must be resolved. Evaluative priorities may not track values if we underestimate or overestimate their importance, or deny their existence. (Faulkner's character in *Absalom, Absalom* fervently repeats to himself "I do not hate the South.") Evaluative priorities may not track goals if we are distracted or forgetful. Unresolved ambivalence will defeat decision making, leaving us suspended between options, like Buridan's ass. And procrastination of various sorts can defeat the whole enterprise by postponing action until it is too late.

However, it is obvious that under duress, self-command also requires courage and persistence. At every point in this process of self-conscious deliberation and agentic activity, we need the strength to resist the efforts of others (or impersonal events in the physical or social environment) to defeat the process. And we need the persistence and endurance to prevail against motivation-draining difficulties.

Finally, self-command can be self-defeating even if it resolves all of these other problems but at the same time lacks a self-correcting feedback loop. Reliably competent functioning must involve a process of assessment and revision through which errors can be corrected and improvements can be made.

Acquisitions, appropriation, attachments, and holdings. Both as an instrument of self-preservation and as part of the development of individual personality, human beings not only define personal boundaries (both physical and psychological) but also make some things their own. The preceding discussions of the circumstances of habilitation and of good health make clear that acquisitive dispositions of some sorts are involved in basic good health in every hospitable environment, since they are always part of self-preservation and self-habilitation. It follows that people in basic good health will also be motivated to modulate their acquisitiveness to avoid self-destructive and self-defeating forms of it.

As noted earlier, the forms of ownership consistent with habilitation differ dramatically from environment to environment. Sometimes this appears to be due to arbitrary social conventions that have successfully solved cooperation and coordination problems and which have become deeply entrenched social practices. But sometimes these differences correspond to nonarbitrary differences in what various physical and social environments require of rational agents—for example, by way of adaptability to changing circumstances, or by way of dealing with a thinly populated, austere physical environment.

So there is no reason to suppose that human beings cannot achieve and sustain basic good health with a wide variety of individual dispositions about acquisitiveness, appropriation, and the resulting individual and even idiosyncratic attachments and holdings. The only general points to be made seem to be that basic good health will entail the presence of some important dispositions of these sorts and will entail having versions of them that permit reliably competent functioning in environments that are accessible to the individuals involved.

This is a commonsensical point, ratified by evidence from economic anthropology, economic history, cultural anthropology and history, and implicitly by developmental psychology as well. But the obviousness of this does not mean that it needs no mention in a book about justice. Such books almost always make property rules central in one way or another, and sometimes by arguing either for or against the "naturalness" of private ownership or various forms of it. The point here is simply that whatever perfect justice may require in the way of uniform property rules that are applicable everywhere, basic good health requires very little uniformity.

Navigable path(s) from basic good health to better forms of well-being and a good life. There is similar diversity in what basic good health entails by way of the healthy individual's conception of well-being and a good life beyond that given by basic good health itself, in an appropriately hospitable environment. One can find the evidence for this, again, in anthropology, history, biography, autobiography, and narrative art. There is simply no reason to believe that basic good health entails any one of the forms of perfect well-being or the best form of life projected by psychological, philosophical, or theological theories. Basically healthy people are physically and psychologically diverse—dramatically so—even within small, tight social structures like families.

What basic good health does seem to entail is for each healthy individual to have at least one navigable path from basic good health to something even better. That kind of progress, involving agency in an essential way, is strongly motivated. When it is utterly impossible—when there is no such navigable path for an individual—the predictable reactions tend to compromise good health. Desperation or inanition can result from feelings of helplessness, being trapped, stunted, blocked, excluded from the possibility of better-than-merely-competent functioning or a better-than-merely-acceptable life. Those things can eventually erode the good health necessary for preventing ill health.

Is more than one navigable path necessary for basic good health? We can probably say that having only one is a threat to basic health to the extent that it might be lost and that the individual involved is unable to adapt—either through rehabilitation which uncovers additional paths, or through a form of acceptance that does not erode health. (One thinks of age as a significant factor here.) But that is just to say that while the lack of alternative paths can be psychologically debilitating, it is not necessarily so for people who are confident of their ability to adapt or are confident of their lack of need to do so.

Idiosyncrasy. This discussion has repeatedly called attention to the diversity of basically healthy personalities. Human endowments, development, surrounding physical and social environments, and activities are complex and varied. Basic good health in any given environment or range of environments is always a range of possibilities rather than a singular, necessary point on the health scale. Idiosyncrasy is abundant.

That is a fact about individuality which presents obvious problems for the intersection of basic good health and basic justice. If idiosyncrasy is to some degree inevitable (and strongly motivated in the sense that it is an inevitable by-product of important forms of habilitation and agentic activity), and if basic justice requires sameness of motivation in many respects, then there is a possible tension. The solution, just in terms of the motivational structure of personality, would be the development of a disposition of tolerance for diversity that can exist with dispositions of justice. This is obviously consonant with something like Mill's principle of liberty, though the details of the harm principle can be expected to vary from environment to environment.

Self-respect. Finally, with respect to individuality, it is worth noting the connection between basic good health and self-respect. There are strong connections, at least once rational agency has developed. Such healthy agents will have an appreciation of their own subjectivity and its uniqueness. They will have developed forms of mutuality that include mutual respect. They will have a vivid appreciation of human diversity and both their own sameness to other humans and their own idiosyncrasy. They will have a sharp sense of both the necessities and possibilities of the habilitative tasks they face and will face throughout their lives—motivating personal demands for necessary goods and protection from necessarily self-destructive and self-defeating things. They will have personal boundaries, attachments, and possessions—motivating additional personal demands. They will demand and protect at least one navigable path to a life they regard as better than the one they have. And they will demand tolerance for their own idiosyncrasies, insofar as they see those as necessary products of their basic good health, and as harmless to others.

This is a strong form, and strongly motivated form, of self-respect. It does not come from metaphysical claims about the infinite worth of rational beings or from ethical claims about the equal worth of persons. It is rather a multifaceted disposition to demand respect from other persons for one's own person, and it is something that develops in a basically healthy personality, in genuinely hospitable environments. And it is another of the heterogeneous motivational elements of personality that basic good health integrates into reliably competent functioning.

2.3. *Cooperation*

Habilitation depends on widespread social cooperation as well as sociality and individuality. Basically healthy rational agents have vivid appreciation of this, as well as the cooperation problem which arises from conflicts within and between persons. Such conflicts do not all arise from Humean circumstances of justice (moderate scarcity, limited altruism, and roughly balanced power and vulnerability). They also arise from the necessity for habilitation into health, and consequently the strongly motivated sources of mutuality, the sometimes conflicting sources of individuality, the conflicting demands of persons, and the ways in which failing to solve cooperation problems (and solve them efficiently) exhausts the energy for and possibilities of the habilitation necessary for health.

So the social cooperation necessary for habilitation into basic health—into reliably competent functioning in a given environment—is strongly motivated in any genuinely hospitable environment and remains so for any individual in basically good health. At least that is so if basically healthy, rational agents can find a way to solve such problems that preserves good health, in the form of a coherent, integrated motivational structure and behavioral dispositions for rational agency.

They cannot always do this, of course. Basic good health does not mean that healthy agents will be perfectly knowledgeable, or that deliberation will be error free. Health does not mean that agents will always be able to avoid fixed beliefs, prejudices, loyalties, and attachments that prevent some kinds of cooperation. And it does not mean that basically healthy rational agents will not sometimes have such fixed beliefs or attachments so deeply entrenched in their personalities that compromising them will be self-defeating psychologically, or even self-destructive. But it does mean that they will continue to have strong motivation toward some sort of solution to cooperative deadlocks, and specifically toward second-order solutions to cooperation problems such as those mentioned later, as long as they are not directly self-destructive or self-defeating.

The question now is simply a matter of identifying the general nature of such habilitative health-creating and health-sustaining solutions. They are not difficult to find, and they have been described too often in the literature on justice to require much elaboration. Here are the leading elements, in no particular order of priority.

Agentic activity and self-command. Agentic activity in which self-command, practical wisdom, and the preservation of navigable options for a better life are present as leading concerns is a necessary good for healthy rational agency. This is true no matter how thoroughly one might be subordinated in a social structure. (Think of the lowest ranking enlisted soldier in the chain of command.) Agency and self-command may be limited dramatically, in some circumstances, without eroding basic good health. But there is a large psychiatric literature on the way in which some social environments systematically undermine, rather than merely limit, agency, and thus erode good health into illness. Rational agents will want to find solutions to cooperation problems which preserve their health as agents.

Possibilities for sufficient cooperation. Agents cooperate in the expectation that enough others will do likewise to make the effort successful. Rational agents assess the possibilities for sufficient cooperation from others, and their certainties or uncertainties about these things have consequences for their motivation. In general, the motivation is strongest when the agent is certain of sufficient cooperation from others; it diminishes (or is complicated) by the certainty that cooperation from others will be insufficient. Futile cooperative activity—or rather the belief that it will be futile—can extinguish it altogether, or complicate it with a form of dogged persistence that is quixotic. People can wash their hands of it and walk away, or clench their teeth and continue a losing effort. This is true of cooperation in dyadic relationships such as a marriage, or larger familial or collegial or commercial ones. It is true of large-scale volunteer efforts and in political participation. It is true in local or national or international politics.

Basic good health will not prevent the breakdown of cooperative activity once the expectation of enough of it from others is extinguished. But it will sustain the motivation to isolate the source of the breakdown as far as possible from other cooperative activities that in themselves remain possible. And it will sustain the motivation to find a way around the breakdown, limit the damage from it, and try again when success seems once more possible. Courage and persistence are as much a part of basic good health as are self-respect, nonnegotiable demands, and attachments.

Deadlocks and second-order solutions. Nonetheless, unresolved deadlocks may remain, with destructive or damaging consequences for good health and for habilitative tasks generally.

Sometimes people are deadlocked in ways that keep them apart (or together), when some form of constructive engagement (or disengagement) is habilitatively necessary. For example, governments may refuse to recognize each other's legitimacy and refuse to negotiate with each other, either directly or indirectly, even to preserve an environment hospitable enough for long-term coexistence. A divorcing couple may separate but give their lawyers instructions that effectively stall the necessary legal proceedings. And then they may refuse direct or indirect negotiations with each other, even to preserve their own long-term economic and psychological well-being. Similar deadlocks occur in neighborhoods, voluntary organizations, bureaucracies, and legislative bodies.

Since basic good health sustains a strong general motivation toward the cooperation necessary for habilitative tasks generally, and away from the destructive or damaging consequences of the failure of such cooperation, it will also motivate second-order solutions to these deadlocks. That is, when the parties involved cannot themselves resolve the deadlock directly, as long as they remain in basically good health they will be motivated to accept, or at least not refuse, a procedure which resolves the deadlock for them. Social conventions can have this effect informally, through peer pressure and a general cooling of social relationships generally. So can shame, or ostracism. Organizational rules can have the same effect more formally, by imposing rules of order on the dispute and imposing procedures for ending it. Legal intervention can impose a decision and enforce it with sanctions.

The remaining questions for the deadlocked parties are whether to submit to such second-order procedures, and then whether to accept the specific resolution they provide. Basic good health will motivate an individual to accept (or at least not to refuse)[5] such second-order procedures and solutions as long as such acceptance is consistent, in the long run, with continued habilitation toward good health and away from self-destructive or self-defeating consequences.

A few things are worth noting about this motivational condition on accepting second-order resolutions of deadlocks. For one, damage to at least one party is inevitable. So the motivational condition cannot be against risking damage of any sort. The deadlock itself risks damage, and it is by hypothesis also strongly motivated. What else could account for its persistence? So the motivational condition on second-order solutions is a relative one, identical to what one expects for direct solutions of the deadlock itself: the damage risked by the solution cannot be greater than the damage risked by continued deadlock, and there must be a greater potential for long-term improvement in well-being from the solution than from the continued deadlock.

For another thing, accepting second-order procedures involves self-command for both parties and the form of self-respect involved in it. So that part is also congruent with the motivation of the deadlock itself. But in addition, the social aspect of second-order solutions involves forms of mutual recognition and respect which implicitly carry a form of mutual honor. This is true even when second-order solutions are invented by the parties themselves and unknown to others, though it is probably increased when the solutions involve social conventions, or even legal proceedings. In any case, this mutuality also supports self-respect for both parties.

Furthermore, simply having the deadlock definitively resolved by second-order "rules" can be dramatically less risky than either continuing the struggle or unilaterally conceding defeat. It gives clarity and predictability to the result, and in many cases brings effective social constraints against reprisals or renewal of hostilities. This, together with simply getting it over with and moving on, is often restorative.

Finally, and most important, the success and availability of second-order solutions to cooperation problems strongly motivate the prospective use of such methods to prevent breakdowns and deadlocks before they arise. We voluntarily assume certain risks (or at least do not refuse them) and accept forms of rehabilitative social insurance (and adjudication of claims) that are already in place. As long as nothing undermines either the voluntary aspect of this or the adequacy of the rehabilitative social insurance, this greatly increases the range and stability of

---

[5] This is an inexact motivational analog to the important distinction, developed by T. M. Scanlon, between reasonable agreement and reasonable nonrefusal (Scanlon, *Utilitarianism and Beyond,* 1982). His full-scale development of that idea is in his book *What We Owe to Each Other* (1998).

the cooperation needed for a genuinely hospitable environment. It also increases the amount of risk people might be motivated to take with respect to their own self-preservation and well-being. This is so because it embeds concerns about one's own immediate well-being in a social matrix of role responsibilities and on-going social responses to damage from them, which can radically alter individual calculations.

Physically and psychologically dangerous activities that are necessary for sustaining (many) hospitable environments provide the best examples when they are coupled with significant forms of social insurance. These include childbearing, certainly, as well as dangerous occupations such as mining, firefighting, police work, and military service. People regularly risk their lives in these activities, and such risk can be strongly motivated by basic good health.

Similarly for many other risky endeavors, even without much in the way of social insurance. For example, the conventional and expectable pattern of conduct of experienced rock climbers typically involves an expected but rare form of self-sacrifice: cutting the rope to prevent your fall from dragging others down with you. It may be prospectively rational to climb under conditions in which you and all your partners are motivated to do this, and not rational otherwise, with or without social insurance.

Predictability. A good deal of the discussion so far has shown that the motivation for cooperation is tied importantly to the predictability of favorable outcomes. We want to know whether we are likely to get sufficient cooperation from others, and whether there are habilitative social structures in place as insurance against failure or damaging outcomes. The same thing is true for every context in which our behavior must be strategic. Predictability helps.

Basic good health, when it is widespread throughout the population, provides broad and powerful forms of motivation for cooperation as well as for the forms of mutuality and individuality already discussed. And more generally, it provides widespread, reliably competent agency throughout the population. Even though there is great diversity in the details of basically healthy personality throughout any population, there are also significant, reliable patterns of motivation and behavior that are characteristic of basic good health. This is of fundamental importance in matters of cooperation, coordination, and conflict resolution. And since cooperation is fundamentally important to creating and sustaining hospitable environments, we have a strong motivation for making sure basic good health is in fact typical of the population at large, insofar as we can do so prospectively without making the effort self-defeating or dystopic.

Additional sources of predictability come from human propensities for routines, repetition, ritual, and other sorts of patterned conduct. These propensities not only help to make our behavior more predictable in itself, but that predictability leads to social expectations and eventually to regularized or institutionalized forms of customary behavior. Such social conventions, including some aspects of etiquette, often also express and reinforce mutual recognition, mutual benevolence, and mutual respect.

Trustworthiness and transparency in cooperative behavior. Cooperative behavior often involves an element of risk for an individual. Predictability can reduce that risk. And the trustworthiness of others not only increases predictability but also sustains and extends the form of basic trust acquired by healthy infants and children in genuinely hospitable environments. It turns basically trusting motivation into reliably competent trusting behavior.

Trustworthiness has at least three leading elements. One is credibility: you are trustworthy in this respect to the extent that it is safe for others to believe what you say. Part of that is that you do not disguise your speculations or unsupported opinions as knowledge. Another part is that what you define as knowledge is something others can recognize as such, and if not, that you make clear that your epistemology is unusual. And a third part of credibility is that you do not lie in ways that put other cooperative people at greater risk because they believe what you say. Dealing with a person who is credible in these ways supports both the motivation for basic trust and its reliably competent functioning with respect to cooperative behavior.

A second element of trustworthiness is reliable agency itself. You are trustworthy to the extent that you are a reliably competent agent in a given environment. Whether you are credible is a separate matter. A person with valuable talents can be trustworthy in this sense even if what he or she actually says is not always credible. (Since stress-induced worry can exacerbate heart problems, part of a cardiologist's competence may be his willingness to be reassuring to his patients well beyond the point of speaking the truth.)

And a third element of trustworthiness is nonmalevolence. You are trustworthy in this sense if it is safe for others to have confidence in the benevolence or at least nonmalevolence of your motives. Whether it is also safe for them to believe what you say and to believe that you are a reliably competent agent are separate issues. But a part of the trust that sustains the motivation for cooperative behavior depends on the confidence that one is not dealing with an enemy. Without that confidence, one is guarded at best and in high-stakes cases may not be willing to cooperate at all.

Transparency. Sustaining the motivation for cooperative behavior often depends upon mutual transparence—about each other's motives, goals, and intentions. This is always a matter of degree, given the limitations of self-knowledge among other things, and is often better described as translucence. And of course in competitive endeavors (commercial transactions, policy negotiations, games) the parties may deliberately conceal a good many things about their strategy and goals. But the overall nature of the endeavor needs to be clear so that the predictability and confidence necessary for cooperation is possible. Reliably competent agents are motivated to get and give the information necessary for cooperation—both by being appropriately transparent and by expecting transparency from others.

Division of labor, and clarity about role responsibilities. The cooperative tasks necessary for habilitation (especially the habilitation of the physical and social environments into genuinely hospitable ones) can be enormously burdensome. Out of concern for avoiding self-destructive and self-defeating activities, individuals are understandably motivated to increase the fit between their own burdens and their own basic good health (including the preservation of a navigable path to even better well-being and a good life). That means, among other things, that a division of labor will be strongly motivated if it can be designed to promote and sustain basic good health by simplifying and distributing burdens toward that end and to increase the efficiency and effectiveness of work through the expertise of specialists.

This motivation for cooperative behavior can be increased still further if it allows people to satisfy what Rawls calls the Aristotelian principle: "human beings enjoy the exercise of their realized capacities, and this enjoyment increases the more the capacity is realized, or the greater its complexity" (Rawls, 1971, 436). And further reinforcement of the motive is supplied by the transparent and predictable patterns of behavior such a division of labor involves, through its clarity about role responsibilities.

Once a division of labor has been arranged—structured so as to sustain basic good health for the individuals involved—and role responsibilities have been clarified, reliably competent agents will be motivated to monitor the way the initial distribution of burdens is continued (or changed) over time. One can expect tension—or even deadlock—between a conservative motive to preserve things as they are (the devil you know) and a progressive motive to risk change that might yield an improvement. And one can expect that various second-order solutions to such tension will also be motivated.

One important sort of second-order solution is to focus on maintaining the consistency of the individual burdens involved rather than on maintaining the actual tasks or role responsibilities themselves. Focusing on predictable consistency of that sort is effectively to focus on "fair play" in the context of an evolving social institution. One is motivated to sign on to a cooperative scheme for certain general reasons (e.g., health and well-being) as well as particular ones (the opportunity to be a village blacksmith). When the need for village blacksmiths diminishes to the vanishing point, what sustains the motivation to continue to cooperate is surely, in large part, the availability of some opportunity that is comparable in terms of its benefits and burdens. As a motivational matter, this becomes especially acute if the disappearance of village blacksmiths has opened up dazzling possibilities for some people but has eliminated all but an assortment of unattractive ones for blacksmiths. In the parlance of justice, blacksmiths are likely to develop a sharp sense of unfairness and injustice in such circumstances unless their general cooperative burdens and benefits can be kept at least roughly consistent with what they had been.

Reciprocity. This brings us to reciprocity. It is a practice, governed by elaborate social norms, in every genuinely hospitable social environment of record. The details of the practice vary widely from one society to another, but they are all elaborations of the same general concept: responses to others for the benefits and burdens one receives from them should be fitting and proportional. They should be fitting in the sense of being of the same general kind—benefits for benefits, for example. They should be proportionate in a way analogous to paying a debt. Both overpayments and underpayments tend to create trouble, even if only by creating something more for the parties involved to deal with before moving on. Excessive or deficient ones are likely to be disturbing enough to one party or the other to make the whole exchange self-defeating. Think of disproportionate punishments. Or even disproportionately generous dinner invitations.

Since reciprocity is a strongly motivated social norm in hospitable social environments generally, that sort of motivation will develop as part of basic good health as well. That is, reliably competent agents will have to be able to cope with it by being disposed to conform to it when it is necessary for the successful pursuit of habilitative tasks. And they will be motivated to adopt a conception of reciprocity—an elaboration of the general concept of it—that is consistent with competent functioning in the environments they inhabit.

This has important consequences for constructing a conception of reciprocity. All of them are connected to the necessity to make reciprocity a behavioral pattern that is productive for habilitation into basic good health. That means it will have to be defined in ways that are not widely destructive of health.

On the benefit-for-benefit side of things, that will require solving the proportionality problem in a way that does not further increase damaging inequalities. The conception of reciprocity must preserve the health of people who are unable, for whatever reason, to return benefits equal in value to the ones they receive.

In such circumstances, an equal benefit interpretation of proportionality can be the source of great inequalities, over time, in power and liberty and health. People who provide benefits at low marginal cost to themselves, and who insist on equal benefits in return even when that exacts a very high marginal cost from others, contribute to a downward spiral of this sort. On those grounds, I have elsewhere argued for an equal marginal sacrifice interpretation of proportionality (Becker, 2005, 26–30).

On the burden-for-burden side of things, basic good health will require a solution to the proportionality problem that is rehabilitative wherever possible. See the discussion of retaliation and punishment in the next chapter.

Additionally, the conception of reciprocity growing out of these concerns for habilitation will emphasize the importance of initiating new reciprocal relationships, restoring damaged ones, and maximizing the predictable and controllable benefits from cooperation and the performance of role responsibilities. In doing so it will help define criteria for basic forms of mutual aid and mutual restraint.

Hospitality, gifts, and rescue. There are other notable forms of mutual aid and mutual restraint that increase predictability as well, as long as they remain in the context of general cooperative and reciprocal conduct. Norms of hospitality, gift giving, and rescue are probably as common as norms of reciprocity in genuinely hospitable social environments. Again, the details vary widely from society to society. And again, the connection to basic health is at least that reliably competent functioning will entail dispositions appropriate to the relevant range of environments.

2.4. *Regulation, damage control, rectification, and retaliation*

The motivational structure of basic good health does not guarantee that people who have that motivational structure will agree with each other about what should be done in particular cases, or how it should be done. Nor does it guarantee that such motivation, even when it is quite strong, will always be determinative for behavior. And of course it is implausible to think that this motivational structure could ever be uniformly distributed throughout the population, at any uniform level of strength. Some people will effectively not have it at all and will be dysfunctionally asocial or antisocial. Others will have almost all of it and will be reliably competent agents in most respects, and competent enough to get away with a significant amount of asocial or antisocial behavior in other respects—though at considerable cost to themselves and others.

It is worth being a little bit more specific about the range of these problems. It is obvious that if they are widespread enough throughout the population they will compromise habilitation, and that the consequences will be severe. It is also obvious that they have always been widespread, and that without effective second-order solutions to these problems of first-order motivation, habilitation is also severely compromised. So basically healthy people, in genuinely hospitable environments, will be strongly motivated to find solutions for the following range of problems.

Occasionally distorted motivation and behavior. People in basically good health can be overwhelmed in particular cases by physical or psychological trauma, confusion, ambivalence, ignorance, self-deception, fear, doubt, desire, or attachment (or the lack of it) in ways that distort their behavior, turning it away from habilitative agentic activity, self-command, mutuality, and cooperation, and turning it instead toward self-destructive or self-defeating ends. Sometimes these distortions lead to downward spirals that eventually become irreparable. Sometimes, also, they spread to others like a contagious disease. Think of the damage that can be done to a family by severe psychological trauma to one member.

Collapse of hospitable environments. When such distorted motivation is long-lasting and widespread in a given population, or simply occurs in people who are unusually powerful or otherwise well-placed to damage others, it can lead to systemic damage. (Think of Stalin, Hitler, Pol Pot.) And when habilitative efforts begin to fail throughout the social environment, the environment itself may become inhospitable or even nonsurvivable. For example, it is plausible to think that rigidity about permissible forms of life and the consequent failure to adapt to changes in the physical environment have sometimes led to the complete collapse of hospitable social environments (Turnbull, 1972; Diamond, 2005; Wilkinson, 2011). Basic good health may then become impossible to develop and sustain.

Global intellectual and motivational impairments. The danger of these distortions of good health in particular cases is multiplied by further factors. One is that every nonfanciful historical account of a multigenerational human community describes a significant population of people for whom basic good health is apparently not achievable, as a practical matter. Or at any rate it is not achieved. Illness does not always touch healthy motivational structure, of course, because it might not be damaging psychologically at all. But when it touches agency directly, and in a global way, it certainly does damage basically healthy motivation.

At the extremes, such cases include profound intellectual impairments (anacephalic infants, profound dementia, persistent vegetative state), and profoundly pathological motivational structures and behaviors, such as those found in psychotic states. But there are people who are profoundly asocial as well, so much so that they cannot function competently as agents at all within a social environment unless they are closely cared for in that environment. Such impairments may take the form of an incapability to engage in any form of social interaction (extreme forms of autism), or incapability to have any form of genuinely mutual interaction with others that involves empathy, and the consequent capability of engaging in almost any kind of asocial antisocial behavior (psychopathy). At any of these extremes, the overall motivational structure is damaged, perhaps irreparably.

Localized damage to sociality. Social environments also typically include a significant population of vigorous, energetic, and otherwise capable agents who do not have the entire repertoire of motivation characteristic of basic good health. Such populations include people who are openly asocial only when it comes to a particular kind of mutuality or cooperation—say, a misanthropic, reclusive Scrooge with minimal, grudgingly reciprocal social connections, or an intensely competitive and domineering person who uses reciprocal relationships in a thoroughly exploitative way. It also includes people who are openly malicious and antisocial in some circumstances (such as an emotionally or physically abusive spouse or parent at home), but benevolent, cooperative, and highly social in others. (How often do neighbors and coworkers say "I never would have guessed. He seemed so nice.")

Free riders, grifters, and professional criminals. Outright concealment of antisocial behavior is another problem. Every society has a population of cheaters, grifters, thieves, and criminals, along with people who deliberately or recklessly harm others and hide their role in doing it. More generally, there are people who take great pains to conceal their unwillingness to cooperate or to reciprocate, or who conceal their antisocial motives and behavior. These people depend upon others' having the motivational structure of basic good health. Free riders need the benefits of others' cooperation and reciprocity. Grifters need gullible marks. Criminals need banks to rob, trustworthy people to defraud, defenseless people to injure or kill. They do not want to be caught. They do not want to have so many other people in their line of work that the banks erect impregnable defenses or that people everywhere guard themselves against fraud and violent crime so that free riding becomes difficult to conceal.

Selective refusal. Finally, there is the problem of selective refusal to cooperate or to work toward second-order solutions. This includes cases in which the only difference between the motivational structure of defectors and cooperators is that the defectors refuse, on a given issue, to consider any alternative to refusal. Their position is implacable, but limited. They will not leave for another social environment, but as a matter of principle they will not contribute toward a certain generally accepted social goal, which they oppose, but which they acknowledge they cannot change. They do not wish to damage others or make the environment less hospitable. They simply opt out, for "personal reasons." Some members of a homeowners association may refuse to pay a special assessment for playground equipment on the common lot. Some members of a university faculty may refuse all departmental committee assignments. Some citizens may refuse to vote or to declare certain sorts of income for tax purposes.

Selective refusal also includes cases of limited secession from the larger social environment—so as to establish a form of life incompatible with that larger environment, but coexistent with it. Think of closed religious communities which have no interest in damaging or subverting the larger societies in which they are embedded. Complete secession, violent or nonviolent, is also a possibility.

But selective refusal also includes conscientious disobedience designed to force changes in a social environment that one does not intend to leave—changes that are meant to improve it. When the changes are big ones and the force involved to get them (or prevent them) is sometimes coercive or violent, this sort of selective refusal becomes revolutionary in its aims. The women's suffrage movement in early twentieth-century England is an example, as is the mid-twentieth-century civil rights movement in the United States.

Vigilance, persistence, and second-order solutions. All of the foregoing problems are stubborn and potentially damaging to habilitative tasks, and thus to basic good health itself. The motivational structure of basic health is strongly oriented away from self-destructive or self-defeating behavior and toward accomplishing the habilitative tasks necessary for sustaining good health. It will not always be possible to translate such motivation into appropriate, effective action. But as long as basic good health is widespread throughout a genuinely hospitable environment, there is good reason to think that even the most stubborn of these problems can be managed so as to at least limit the damage.

The resources available are obvious. The motivational structure of basic good health would put considerable pressure on people to be vigilant about identifying and correcting their own deficiencies in agentic activity (including ignorance, self-deception, errors about what is necessary and possible, and their ability to translate careful deliberation into appropriate judgments and conduct). It would also make them persistent about pursuing solutions to cooperation problems and directing a good deal of habilitative activity toward preventing them from arising in the first place. That persistence would generate continual pressure to widen the extent of the population for whom basic good health is possible and to minimize the extent to which the distribution of benefits and burdens of cooperative activity systematically undermine basic good health.

8

Healthy Agency and the Norms of Basic Justice

The discussion now turns to the interesting parallels between the motivational structure characteristic of basic health, as discussed in Chapter 7, and the norms of basic justice. It is clear enough at this point that basic good health will include a wide range of stable and strongly motivated dispositions *about* the subject matter of basic justice. And it is clear enough that such behavioral dispositions could in principle be represented as embodiments of stable and strongly motivated norms *of* justice. After all, habilitative necessities, possibilities, and impossibilities can be expressed in the language of normative requirements, possibilities, and prohibitions. And if their subject matter overlaps with the subject matter of basic justice, to say that the norms of justice are stably and strongly motivated for people in basically good health is to say that people can understand their motivations *about* justice as norms *of* justice.

But does the motivational structure of basic health parallel *all* the norms of basic justice in this way? The two will certainly diverge in one important way: basically healthy people are strongly motivated toward self-preservation and away from self-destructive and self-defeating conduct, even when they cannot, as a matter of justice, effectively *require* of themselves and others that all such things be accomplished. The best basic justice can do is to manage things within our limited possibilities. As a result, there will not be a one-to-one mapping of the entirety of basically healthy motivation onto the norms of basic justice. At best there will be a one-to-one mapping within some partial intersection of the two. Even so, getting clear about the extent of that intersection is not easy.

The initial difficulty is that we do not have a *detailed* description of items on either side of the equation. Nor is it plausible to think we could get such lists. What is motivated as habilitative necessity, for example, varies dramatically from one range of hospitable environments to another. Life in a thinly populated and precarious physical environment will not be able to tolerate much in the way of defection from necessary cooperative tasks. It will put a premium on physical vigor and strength, and not much on the exacting communication and coordination required for life and work in a large, contemporary urban environment. It is unclear, a priori, whether the details of the norms of justice will reflect those differences in habilitative necessities.

So for present purposes, the best we can do in lining up the motivational and behavioral dispositions of basic good health with the norms of basic justice is to ask (1) whether there is a one-to-one mapping of large general categories of items on each side of the equation, (2) whether there are no obvious items or general categories on those lists that contradict each other, except in their details, and (3) whether, as we attempt to construct a more detailed list on one side of the equation, we find that comparable items emerge on the other side.

In all of this, however, there is another difficulty. Although the subject matter of basic justice is clear enough in historical practice and philosophical theory, its normative content has not previously been described (as far as I am aware) in terms designed to show its connection to the motivational and dispositional content of basic good health. So my account here will be a reconstruction, the success of which will depend upon not going beyond, or otherwise distorting, the general normative content of basic justice as it is more typically described—for example, in terms of elements that are found in legal and social norms within hospitable social environments everywhere.

This reconstruction of the norms of justice is meant to be descriptive. And although any reconstruction of this sort is done conceptually rather than empirically, this one aims to remain close to the data-driven parts of comparative anthropology, comparative legal and social history, analytical and comparative jurisprudence, and related areas of economics, political science, psychology, and sociology.

1. Habilitative Necessities and Justice

The most fundamental connection between basic health and basic justice is through the identification of habilitative necessities for human beings within a given environment. This matches the most fundamental self-preservative and self-protective dispositions of basic good health with comparable norms of basic justice.

Population health: sufficiency norms. The task of working toward and maintaining a genuinely hospitable environment depends upon making sure that basic good health, and especially healthy agency, is widespread enough across a multigenerational population to ensure the success of such habilitative efforts. And it is clear enough that normative requirements along this line are part of the consensus defined by basic justice. This is reflected in the prominence of concerns in every social group about the existence and distribution of the things necessary for individual and population health. Whether health itself is specifically discussed or not, the things necessary for it certainly are: for example, the physical resources necessary for nutrition and physical vigor; the courage, persistence, self-command, and productive work necessary for securing those resources. The same virtues apply to reproductive work, care of the young, and education. All of these things have always been central concerns of distributive justice.

The consensus about population health that we can expect at the level of basic justice is for (1) the prohibition of distributive schemes that make it impossible to have enough individuals in basically good health to create, sustain, or restore the genuinely hospitable nature of the social environment; (2) the requirement for a distributive scheme that guarantees the things necessary for basic good health to a wide enough range of individuals to produce (in favorable circumstances) enough healthy individuals to make it possible to sustain or restore the genuinely hospitable nature of the social environment.

There are two limitations on these norms of basic justice that pose problems and opportunities for full-scale theories of distributive justice. One is that consensus on more strongly progressive norms for population health is blocked by the seemingly perpetual conflict between conservative and progressive attitudes. Even though habilitation toward improvements in individual well-being and the physical and social environment is strongly motivated in basically healthy individuals, there is disagreement about a *requirement* to go beyond what is strictly necessary for habilitation. Doing what is necessary to sustain what we have is one thing; requiring that we make good things better is another. People who focus mostly on preventing bad things from happening tend to treat unnecessary improvements as supererogatory. People who focus mostly on making good things happen sometimes treat such progress as a requirement.

The other limitation of basic justice in these matters is that consensus on the equal distribution of the things necessary for basic good health is often blocked by the discord between hierarchical and relatively nonhierarchical social arrangements. In nonhierarchical arrangements, one is likely to find egalitarian norms of distribution for essential goods, since they operate with at least a rebuttable presumption of equal moral worth. In hierarchical arrangements, by contrast, priorities tend to be skewed toward those at the top of the hierarchy, since their health and well-being is regarded as more important, or more deserved. (Think of what goes to the elite in such societies as opposed to what goes to slaves, or the poor, or the women, or noncitizens, or nonparty members. It is not that the elite want others to be *un*healthy. After all, their talents and labor are valuable. But the elite sometimes worry about others being too healthy to remain compliant—too intelligent, too resourceful, too courageous. And in any case, when resources are scarce, the elite think of their own health as the first priority. Read about the debates from the ancient Roman Senate about the dangers posed by slaves. Reflect on what is known about the allocation of food in present-day North Korea.)

Nonetheless, any initial distribution of the necessities for basic good health is likely to put constant pressure on the norms of basic justice to move toward an equal distribution of those necessities. The reasons for that are cumulative, as follows.

Individual health: sufficiency norms. People in basically good health are strongly motivated toward self-preservation and away from self-destructive or self-defeating conduct. They are persistent, resourceful, and courageous in pursuing those goals. And they pursue them not only for themselves but on behalf of those to whom they are strongly attached, psychologically. Such goals reflect one of the circumstances of habilitation—namely, that basically healthy human beings are more likely to be disposed to adopt patterns of radiating benevolence (reflecting the radiating strength of their attachments) than to adopt patterns of impartial, universal benevolence. And the same is true of most unhealthy human beings as well. It takes very specific circumstances of futility or very specific deformations of health to extinguish the goals rooted in self-preservation and psychological attachment to others.

The stable belief that basic good health itself is necessary for the pursuit of those goals generates persistent demands (by healthy as well as many unhealthy individuals) for the things actually sufficient for basic good health, insofar as they are accessible, for themselves and others to whom they are attached. That includes not only the things necessary for good health but also for things that increase the probability that it can be achieved and sustained. Less than that will not be regarded as normatively sufficient.

The corresponding norm of basic justice with respect to individual health will therefore be stated in terms of sufficiency and possibility: it will be *the requirement for the level of habilitation and rehabilitation sufficient to produce basic good health, insofar as that is possible.* And it is plausible to think that basic justice contains that norm. The remaining question will be about the extent to which that norm applies equally throughout the population. In favorable circumstances it is likely to move (slowly, perhaps) toward increasingly egalitarian formulations, as follows.

Consider a hierarchical society in which the distribution of the things necessary for basically good health is skewed toward the elite. And suppose that skewing is propped up by an inegalitarian theory of justice. But all basically healthy individuals, not just those who are members of the elite, are going to be persistent in working toward the sufficiency goals of basic good health for themselves and for others to whom they are attached. And in reasonably hospitable environments, there will be a natural increase in the population of basically healthy individuals, both among the elite and non-elite, and thus in the overlapping circles of people to whom they are attached and for whose health they also persist in their habilitative efforts. That will result in persistent pressure to reformulate the inegalitarian norms to include a wider and wider segment of the population, even if those norms are effectively propagated by members of the elite.

Insofar as the elite believe that their own health and well-being depend upon the existence of an increasing population of basically healthy individuals outside their ranks, the reformulated distributive norms are likely to reflect that necessity. And in favorable circumstances, this creates a ratchet effect. That effect can then be amplified by increased production of the things necessary for basic good health and by increasing, and increasingly general, unwillingness to accept an inegalitarian distribution of those things.

In unfavorable circumstances, of course, inegalitarian norms can harden rather than soften, and the population of people in basically good health can shrink. But that situation is made less likely by other habilitative necessities.

Individual freedom: necessary forms of agentic autonomy. One of these necessities is individual freedom. To the extent that a genuinely hospitable social environment depends upon the autonomous activity of healthy agents, those agents will require the freedom necessary for such activity. Habilitation into healthy agency always requires considerable self-habilitation and thus considerable freedom for individuals, not only as they develop their agency but also as they subsequently exercise it. Some of that agency is strongly motivated toward acquisition—securing those things necessary for habilitation for oneself and those to whom one is attached. Healthy agency can be damaged or even extinguished when it cannot be exercised in this way and in other ways necessary for self-habilitation. The physical analog is muscle atrophy from disuse.

So it is not surprising to find norms of basic justice that require at least some significant level of individual liberty (including liberty for economic activity and property acquisition) for at least some individuals. It is not surprising to find that the amount of individual liberty involved will vary with the extent of healthy agency required throughout each population to sustain the particular environment at issue. As noted previously, the extent of healthy agency required is always considerable and tends to expand as the social environment expands in size and complexity.

That does not mean that the norms of justice with respect to individual liberty found in tightly controlled totalitarian regimes will be very similar to the norms found in liberal democracies. But if such social environments are genuinely hospitable, and thus able to sustain themselves in a multigenerational community, they will require at least the extent of individual liberty *necessary* for sustaining themselves. They may also require the extent necessary for promoting additional stability, strength, and efficiency in the social environment. I will return to that issue in Section 2.

Cooperation: Necessary forms of mutual restraint and mutual aid. Pursuing habilitative necessities in a hospitable social environment requires cooperation. Some of this is in the form of mutual restraint, and some in the form of mutual aid.

Basic justice includes norms of those sorts, matched by corresponding dispositions in basic good health.

In hospitable social environments we find norms of basic justice prohibiting harm or injury to the health of (some) persons and prohibiting damage to the hospitable nature of the physical or social environment itself. The norms make exceptions for harms, injury, or damage that is itself necessary for self-preservation or self-protection, either at the individual or collective level, and they make exceptions for (or special arrangements for) unintended or unavoidable harms or damage. This corresponds to healthy dispositions to avoid self-destructive or self-defeating behavior and to avoid the sort of intellectual and emotional rigidity that undermines the adaptability necessary for survival in changed circumstances. The cooperation necessary to prohibit such harms is a habilitative necessity to the extent that some level of individual and population health is a similar necessity.

The habilitation provided by some to others is a form of mutual aid in any multigenerational society. Those who habilitate infants and children, and rehabilitate people whose health has been damaged, provide services essential to maintaining a necessary level of population health. Norms of basic justice include requirements for these habilitative necessities, and they are consistent with the motivational structure of healthy agency, though that motivational structure goes well beyond these necessities, as discussed below in Section 3.2.

Cooperation: Necessary forms of role responsibility. A division of labor and clarity about role responsibilities is also characteristic of social environments everywhere and is expressed in norms of justice. Although the details vary greatly from one social environment to another, coordination and cooperation problems with respect to the division of labor must be solved, since no one person can do everything that is necessary. As long as these role responsibilities are consistent with individual health and habilitative necessities generally, they are consistent with the motivational structure of basic good health.

2. Habilitative Stability, Strength, and Efficiency

A genuinely hospitable social environment will be stable with respect to habilitative necessities, which will mean that it will have norms that address such stability. Stability is also linked to the strength of the social environment to resist damage and to recover from it, as well as from habilitation-enhancing efficiencies that are only temporarily advantageous. Most of the norms of basic justice dealing with these matters have to do with managing the tensions between cooperation and individuality, and with stabilizing the forms of mutual restraint and mutual aid necessary for habilitation.

Healthy agency includes a heterogeneous constellation of dispositions toward both cooperation and individuality as well as toward managing the tensions and outright conflict between those motivational elements. It will thus be at least consistent with norms of justice that address these matters if and only if they reflect the habilitative necessities for basic good health, including healthy agency.

As a reminder, recall that to be consistent with good health, the norms of basic justice would have to reflect dispositions toward cooperation, mutual restraint, and mutual aid appropriate to the environment. They would have to reflect dispositions toward mutual recognition and mutual respect; dispositions toward a level of basic trust appropriate to the environment; a disposition of radiating benevolence that results in a general readiness to help others. And, through a process of attachment or appropriation, such norms would have to reflect a disposition to attend to the welfare of (some) others as if it were one's own—resulting, in particular cases, in a readiness to sacrifice one's own welfare on their behalf, much as one would sacrifice a part of one's own welfare in order to protect or advance the rest. And to be consistent with good health, the norms of basic justice would have to reflect its dispositions toward individuality—toward individual good health, self-preservation, self-defense, individual agentic activity and the individual liberty necessary for it, and the pursuit of forms of well-being and a good life beyond merely what is necessary for habilitation into basic good health.

It is again fairly easy to see a large overlap between the motivational structure and behavioral dispositions of healthy agency and the norms of *basic* justice. It is of course all too obvious that historically, the norms of justice in many societies have been inconsistent with widespread good health throughout the population (especially the health of women, slaves, the poor, or those of low social status generally). But insofar as those norms are not now *everywhere* norms of justice (in genuinely hospitable environments), they are not *now* norms of basic justice, even if they once were.

Quite a few of those norms can be grouped under the heading of fairness, and perhaps all of them can be forced into that category. After all, if fairness were a habilitative necessity, human history would have been very different. Instead, when fairness is made normative in a social environment, it seems to be a stabilizing and strengthening factor, in ways that also make the environment more efficient. But historically, it has often operated as a destabilizing motivation as well. Beliefs about unfairness are transformed into convictions that a given society is, in practice, unjust in a very basic way, no matter what norms about habilitative necessities it might have.

Rule-oriented norms of fairness. One source of such beliefs about unfairness has to do with the requirement to make sure the norms of basic justice are administered in terms of general rules and principles. This has a number of important consequences for the habilitative stability, strength, and efficiency of the social environment.

The requirement to treat similar cases similarly, for example, is a formal aspect of practical reasoning, abstracted from particular cases into a general rule of deliberation. If some line of reasoning is adequate to support a decision in one case, then it is adequate to support a relevantly similar decision in relevantly similar cases, absent countervailing reasons to the contrary. Practical reasoning is a strongly motivated element of healthy agency, and the similar cases rule is so generally embedded in norms of justice that it is sometimes called "the" rule of justice.

Other rule-oriented features of fairness also exhibit strong connections to the stability and efficiency of practical reasoning and agentic activity. To the extent that requirements of conduct are imposed case-by-case rather than by general rules, deliberation must also be case-by-case, and devoted in part to predicting what the requirements will be rather than how to meet them. Rules and general principles covering a clear range of cases make requirements more predictable, as long as they are stable and clear in their application, and available in advance. Basic justice is rule-oriented in this way—though various eccentric social arrangements may not be.

This rule- and principle-oriented aspect of fairness has been described as natural justice (D'Entreves, 1964), the minimum necessary content of law (Hart, 1961, 189–195), or the inner morality of law (Fuller, 1964). And it is amply motivated by healthy agency.

Norms of fairness in reciprocity. As noted at several points in the text, a widespread practice of reciprocity exists in every society of record. Though this general practice differs widely in its details from society to society, its general form can be represented in the following two-part norm: (1) People are expected, and sometimes required, to respond fairly and cooperatively to the benefits they receive from others by making a fitting and proportional return of benefits, either to them directly, or through some practice which benefits the community generally. (2) People are permitted, and sometimes expected or required, to respond in fitting and proportional ways to the harms they suffer from others, either directly, or through some social or legal institution.

As a norm of fairness, however, reciprocity is typically constrained by the recognition of the unfairness or injustice of self-destructive or self-defeating interpretations of the notions of fitting and proportional responses. (Children, for example, are not expected to immediately return benefits exactly equal to those received from adults. A simple thank you might suffice. And people are expected to avoid punishing wrongdoers in ways that exacerbate the original harms.)

All of this nicely matches the motivational structure of basic good health. The discussion will come back to part (2). But here we can simply point out that the motivation for part (1), when it is accurately reflected in the norms of basic justice, stabilizes and strengthens cooperation. And to the extent that the norm of reciprocity allows some level of individual control over the required extent of the cooperation driven by it, the practice of reciprocity stabilizes and strengthens individual autonomy as well. It can do that to the extent that it allows people to opt out of initiating reciprocal exchanges.

Norms of role responsibility. A division of labor with a consequent assignment of role responsibilities is also characteristic of social environments everywhere, and when it conforms to norms of fairness and reciprocity, it is a norm of basic justice. Roles determined solely by physical and psychological endowments are not inevitable social "assignments" unless we can do something to change those endowments. For example, if we cannot, as a practical matter, change male and female roles in childbearing—by adding in vitro gestation to in vitro fertilization—then childbearing is not a social assignment. Being the primary caregiver for infants, however, is a social role assignment.

Role responsibilities help to define the kinds and extent of cooperative behavior that are required from people in a given environment. To the extent that they are clear, fair, and reciprocal they contribute to the stability, strength, and efficiency of agentic activity by making requirements and opportunities predictable.

Norms of status. Basic justice has many norms based on status, even in relatively nonhierarchical social environments. Parents and children have some duties just because of their status as parents and/or children. Parents have duties of care, especially for infants and young children, which decrease over time if the children remain basically healthy; young children have duties of reciprocity and compliance, which decrease over time if they remain basically healthy. Siblings have status duties as well. Such familial status duties include duties of mutual restraint (e.g., the prohibition of incest) and mutual aid.

These are "natural" duties in the sense that they depend on status and capability rather than choice and capability. And the status involved can be as general as human being (human rights and duties) or as particular as citizen, neighbor, colleague, or relative. Even when we can later opt out of a particular status acquired at birth, such as citizen, we have duties before we are fully competent to choose the status. And even when we acquire a particular status by choice, such as spouse, friend, or neighbor, we may nonetheless have lingering duties even after we opt out of the relationship. (Think of do's and don'ts involved in going, or not going, to the wedding or funeral of a former spouse.)

Some of these status duties—including parental duties of care, the prohibition of incest, the obligations of citizens—are clearly norms of basic justice. They are not always habilitative necessities, since there are typically alternatives available— for example, to children whose parents abandon them. But they are certainly stabilizing and strengthening factors, and often efficient ones as well. As long as they are consistent with habilitative necessities as well as fairness and reciprocity, they will be consistent with the motivational structure and behavioral dispositions of healthy agency.

Norms of economic activity and property. Individual freedom for agentic activity, including freedom for acquisitive economic activity, is described in the previous chapter as a habilitative necessity. The type and extent that is necessary, however, varies so much from one social environment to another that it is not possible to conclude that a particular form of economic organization is the only one consistent with healthy agency. But there is obviously no consensus in basic justice on this matter either. Rather, the consensus is for having norms for economic activity, property acquisition, and ownership that stabilize and strengthen any given hospitable social environment and make it efficient. The motivational structure and behavioral dispositions of healthy agency will be consistent with such norms as long as they are consistent with rule-oriented fairness, reciprocity, and other norms of cooperation and voluntary obligation.

Rescue and hospitality. The consensus about norms of rescue in basic justice are fairly minimal. In some social environments there is a positive, legal duty to rescue people in danger or distress—and one that does not depend on any special status other than being in the right place at the right time with the right abilities, and which does not depend on any special prior voluntary agreements. In other social environments there is no such legal duty, and in fact there are legal obstacles to such rescue—such as legal liabilities for the inadvertent damage the rescue attempt may cause. In some such social environments, requirements of hospitality are subsumed under duties of rescue, which has the consequence of making them equally minimal.

So the norm about rescue and hospitality in basic justice is probably no more than this: (1) People who have a relevant status or contractual duty to rescue or offer hospitality are required to do so, as long as the attempt does not put them in comparable danger. (2) People without such status or contractual duties are permitted, rather than required, to attempt rescue or offer hospitality, if they have the ability to do so without further endangering the person.

Basic good health will dispose people to do more than that, given the nature and extent of the sociality involved in it, and under favorable conditions, it may push basic justice in the direction of requiring more than it now does.

Norms of voluntary obligation. A great deal of social life is organized in terms of ad hoc, more or less local agreements—ranging from implicit understandings to explicit contracts. Lack of clarity and predictability as well lack of fairness and reciprocity play a role in these sorts of arrangements. But voluntary obligations are so useful for the stability, strength, and efficiency of the smooth functioning of the social environment, and so damaging to those things when people feel unfairly burdened by them, that it is not surprising to find norms about them in basic justice.

Stated generally, the relevant norms of basic justice appear to be these: (1) competent agents may make voluntary agreements with each other which create requirements for their conduct if they are mutually advantageous when made; and (2) in any particular case, unresolved disputes about the competency of the agents involved, the existence and voluntariness of the alleged agreements, or the persistence of mutual advantage nullifies the attempt to create the voluntary obligations at issue. (But see the later discussion of second-order rules.)

Social environments (including developed legal systems) vary so widely about the details that it seems unlikely that they all converge on anything more concrete than that. Even so, the importance of such voluntary obligations is evident. And as long as they are consistent with habilitative necessities, fairness, and reciprocity, they will be consistent with the motivational structure and behavioral dispositions of healthy agency.

Norms of predictability. The habilitative stability, strength, and efficiency of the social environment is greatly enhanced by factors that increase the predictability of social interactions. So for that reason among others, basic justice includes a constellation of norms that have that effect. They define expectable levels of transparency, honesty, credibility, reliability, and nonmalevolence to be found in the agents of a given environment. Thus these norms support the reliably competent functioning of agentic deliberation and choice in a given strategic environment and are consistent with healthy agency.

Civility. Stable, sustainable, and efficient social relationships depend upon maintaining the civility of such relationships. One wants to say more than this, since basic good health certainly motivates more. It motivates mutual recognition, mutual respect and honor, self-respect, and even a certain level of conviviality, all of which contribute to the stability, strength, and efficiency of social interactions.

The consensus norms that characterize basic justice, however, seem much more grudging. Societies differ about requiring anything more than civility as a matter of justice—and the norms of civility are regularly violated (in some social environments) in political debate and with respect to outcasts, criminals, people who do not speak the local language, people with serious disabilities, and so on.

Surprisingly, the best one can probably say concerning the consensus norms about civility that characterize basic justice is something like this: civility in speech and behavior toward others is required in face-to-face interactions unless there is an exception for carrying out one's status or role obligations, but it is not required in indirect interactions unless it would be so egregious as to cause serious harm to a robustly healthy individual of the target's age, in the given social context. This is probably enough to regulate seriously damaging reputation effects, for example, such as the suicide of a teenager subjected to vicious verbal attacks on a blog seen by her peers. But it is certainly not enough to regulate the online comments section following news items.

Again, basic good health motivates more than basic justice requires.

3. Second-order Norms

In *The Concept of Law*, H. L. A. Hart distinguishes primary, duty-imposing rules from secondary rules that identify, legislate, administer, and adjudicate the primary ones. His distinction can be extended to norms of justice, at least with respect to enforcing them and adjudicating disputes about them.

Legitimation. The most fundamental second-order norm is what Hart called the rule of recognition. More generally, it is a settled practice for distinguishing genuine norms from those that are only alleged to be genuine. There is no consensus in basic justice as to what that practice must be, in detail. But there is consensus that there must be such a practice, that it must be consistent with the rule-oriented norms of fairness, and that it must be generally accepted to the extent sufficient to effectively settle questions about which norms are legitimate or genuine. This seems compatible with the dispositions of basic good health.

Dispute resolution. Disputes still arise, of course, even when questions about the legitimacy of given norms has been settled. Matters of fairness and reciprocity may seem to collide with other primary duties or obligations, for example. Unresolved disputes reduce the stability, strength, and efficiency of the social environment, and in extreme cases they can threaten its survival as a hospitable environment. It is thus understandable that the norms of basic justice include some second-order norms about dispute resolution.

The details vary, but the general form seems to be something like this: parties to such disputes are required either to end them by mutual consent or to submit their dispute to a decision-making process (arbitration or adjudication), the results of which they are required to accept.

The discussion of healthy agency includes a discussion of the role of second-order solutions to deadlocks between healthy agents, so again this aspect of basic justice is consistent with basic health. The same is true of the adjudication process itself.

Adjudication. The norms of basic justice with respect to the decision-making processes of arbitration and adjudication include the rule-oriented norms of fairness mentioned earlier, but with some additions. There is a requirement of disinterested adjudication, for example. There is a requirement of "legality" or legitimacy—that decisions appeal only to genuine or legitimate norms. There is the requirement that decisions be nonarbitrary—that there is a reasoned basis for them in the legitimate norms appealed to. There is the requirement that this reasoned basis for judgment be made public, whenever that is necessary to give people advance notice for future conduct. And there is the requirement that at some point this process of adjudication in each particular case must be final and binding on the parties, to the extent that compliance can be enforced and noncompliance can be punished. Again, nothing here seems inconsistent with basic good health.

Enforcement. The requirements, permissions, and prohibitions of basic justice are coupled with methods to ensure compliance. These are defined by second-order norms and range from deterrent social or legal pressure all the way to the formal, legal imposition of sanctions after the fact. It has already been noted that healthy agents will be aware of the necessity for cooperation and compliance with the norms of justice to the level sufficient for accomplishing habilitative tasks. And it has been noted that healthy agents will be vigilant about identifying and responding appropriately to the full range of destructive behavior exhibited by others—both in terms of covert and overt antisocial and asocial behavior. Very low levels of opting out, free riding, fraud, nonviolent crime, and property crime that does not harm individuals may not threaten an otherwise stable and strong hospitable social environment—or be more than a passing annoyance or inconvenience of fear for healthy agents. But there is clearly a tipping point in each case.

The tipping point for basic justice is likely to be lower than the one for basic health. There does seem to be a consensus that "trivialities" need not be pursued as a matter of justice. But there is nonetheless a deontic element in basic justice which puts the threshold of triviality quite low. The law is the law; petty crimes are crimes nonetheless, and though we may not actively chasing you down, if we catch you, you will pay.

For basic health, the tipping point for enforcement is more complex. Second-order enforcement norms will be consistent with the motivational structure and behavioral dispositions of basic health if and only if they are consistent with habilitative necessities as well as healthy dispositions toward fairness and reciprocity. And all of this needs to be seen in the context of keeping these efforts to maintain compliance and punish noncompliance away from practices that are self-destructive or self-defeating for a hospitable environment.

Punishment. This is even more true for punishment that is primarily retributive. The retaliative side of the reciprocity norm addresses some of the motivational concerns about punishment. It directs us to make a fitting and proportional response to the harms and injuries we receive from others. If noncompliance has been harmless except for encouraging more of the same, then a proportionate response must be limited to an otherwise harmless deterrent—such as making the noncompliance public, along with a public threat of sanctions for harmful noncompliance. And a fitting response, presumably, will be one which has an appropriate corrective effect on the noncompliant person rather than one which reinforces noncompliant behavior. And all of this must be consistent with the norms of rule-oriented fairness, including its similar cases rule and advance notice rule.

It is not clear that the norms of basic justice that govern retaliation and punishment are fully consistent with the motivational structure and behavioral dispositions of healthy agents. Those healthy dispositions are generally forward-looking, and focused on habilitative necessities, stability, strength, and efficiency. They are of course consistent with norms of self-protection and self-defense. Healthy agents will resist, violently if necessary, crimes against themselves or against their hospitable environments. And they will be disposed to use sanctions or the threat of sanctions, if necessary, to get sufficient compliance with the norms for habilitative necessities, stability, and strength.

But punishment is another matter. As noted, healthy dispositions toward retaliation are constrained to fitting and proportional punishments that have an appropriate corrective effect (or at least do not have a self-defeating habilitative effect) and are constrained as well by norms of rule-oriented fairness. It is not clear that there is a consensus on anything approaching this in basic justice.

In fact, it may be that basic justice has no substantial consensus about retributive norms at all. Social environments may differ too dramatically on what Hart called the general justifying aim of punishment (1968, 8–11) to support the formulation of even a very general norm about punishment consistent with the healthy dispositions described earlier. Historically, some societies have remained stable for lengthy periods even though they practiced vendettas to an extent that should have been destabilizing and was clearly inconsistent with healthy agency as described here (Elster, 1990). After World War II, the Allied forces conducted the Nuremberg trials, obtaining criminal convictions and harsh punishments which, to some, either clearly violated a fundamental tenet of the rule of law in both the Allied countries and in Germany—namely, the prohibition of ex post facto legislation—or else illegitimately imported principles of morality into systems of positive law (Hart, 1958). To others, there were no such violations, but rather an appeal to principles which everyone involved knew, or should have known, were implicit in positive law (Fuller, 1958). Retribution has constitutional protection in the United States as one of several independent elements of justifiable state interest in defining and administering punishment, and political discourse is often harshly supportive of retribution for its own sake. And of course the harsh treatment of captives in the wake of Al Qaeda's attack on September 11,

2001, which continued for years afterward with very little effective opposition (and quite a lot of effective retributive rhetoric) is another example of the distance between the way retributive norms might look in basic justice and the way retributive motives function in basically healthy agency.

4. Moving beyond Basic Justice

This leads to a final point for this chapter, which can now be made very briefly. Basic good health includes strong motivational elements about basic justice, as well as about levels of well-being and a good life which extend beyond both basic health and basic justice. These will likely have some consequences for the development of basic justice, and thus for full-fledged theories of justice.

Some of those motivational elements of basic good health concern retribution. As just noted, healthy agents will be motivated to make retribution serve habilitative goals. To the extent that basic justice does not now reflect a consensus consistent with that motivation, basic good health will exert developmental pressure on it to do so. That sort of developmental pressure can be expected quite generally whenever people in basically good health are motivated to push against the boundaries of the contemporary consensus about justice. Sometimes this pressure will be toward reducing the diversity of forms of social life permitted by basic justice, as in the case of retribution. And sometimes it will be toward expanding the scope of basic justice to include additional norms, as in the case of access to the things necessary for basic good health. The concluding remarks in Chapter 10 will have more to say about these matters.

Part 4

Relevance, Influence, and Prejudice Revisited

Preface to Part Four

These brief concluding chapters summarize the state of the argument by responding to some remaining objections. Chapter 9 begins with reminders about what has been done, or at least intended, and what has deliberately been left undone. It then makes some additional arguments about the comprehensiveness of the habilitation framework and the adequacy of basic good health as the representative good for basic justice. Chapter 10 takes leave of the project by reconsidering some especially troublesome thoughts about it.

In the years that earlier versions of the manuscript have been circulating, some interested readers have continued to press for less of what is here and more of what is not. Less about habilitation and health; more about the normative import of all of this. In short, they want a normative theory—or at least an endorsement of some specific distributive principles. Why not? they may say. Do you expect that robustly healthy agents will simply, by that fact, *be* basically just? (Well, no.) Do you expect that any society will ever be able to produce robust health in all, or nearly all, of its members? (Well, probably not.) So what do you expect to get out of this habilitation framework, then, and this emphasis on robustly healthy agency? (Well, some significant improvement on what we have.) Some improvements in a specific type of theory of justice? (No. An improvement in theory-building materials.) And that's enough? (Yes.)

The end of that exchange is where these concluding chapters start. They end with a reiteration of its final affirmation. Yes, that's enough.

9

Relevance, Influence, and Prejudice

The arguments for the proposals throughout this book are meant to be relevant to the construction of all plausible, full-scale philosophical theories of justice, but not to be prejudicial to any. That means that whatever influence these proposals may have on those theories should be on their theory-building materials. It should not be an outright endorsement or repudiation of any of their fundamental normative principles and goals.

It also means that there is a particularly important burden of proof on the arguments for these proposals: namely, affirmatively establishing that habilitation into healthy agency is a reasonably comprehensive framework for approaching the subject of basic (distributive) justice. This burden of proof has been addressed in previous chapters, but there are some remainders—some matters that need additional emphasis, some that need additional exposition, and some additional types of objections that need to be answered.

1. Exclusionary Reminders

It is important to return briefly to the general concept of basic justice given in Chapter 1. That general concept establishes criteria of relevance for the discussion of possible objections to the habilitation framework.

Constraints imposed by the general concept of basic justice. First, under the general concept of basic justice used here, the norms of justice have to do with enforceable, practicable, social, or political goals for human conduct that can be given a justification that is accessible to, and in principle acceptable by, all moral agents within a given society, regardless of their religious faith or other ultimate commitments. So a theory-independent framework for theories of *basic* justice should not be expected to address normative issues outside those confines, even though such issues may be of crucial importance to what Rawls calls a comprehensive conception of the good, including a complete conception of a good life, or of the complete or ideal form of life, and justice.

And the general concept implicitly adds a further constraint: that these norms and the arguments for and against them must be accessible to moral agents everywhere, just as we expect this of science and mathematics. This excludes all frameworks that rely exclusively on an esoteric epistemology—one that is accessible only to a closed circle of initiates. We can imagine a situation in which many moral agents are interested primarily in whether or not their own esoteric epistemology justifies various norms of justice. But in that case, the framework and metric for basic justice must still be drawn from what Rawls calls the overlapping consensus about justice among moral agents everywhere. The habilitation framework will meet that test if it is drawn from common ground.

Distributive questions within an existing social environment. Second, it is worth noting that the habilitation framework is offered here for distributive questions that arise *within* an ongoing social and political environment—local, national, or international. The basic design of an ideal constitutional system as well as ideals about membership in it are outside the scope of my concerns here. Those are obviously matters of justice, and the habilitation framework is relevant to them. (It is not uncommon, for example, for defenders of a particular kind of social or political system to argue that it is ultimately the healthiest form of social or political life for human beings.) But the argument here is not about ideal justice. The habilitation framework may be the best one, or at least an adequate one, for thinking through those issues also. But that is outside the scope of this book.

Basic distributive questions, not detailed corrective ones. Third, the project here also postpones some questions about corrective, as opposed to distributive, justice. For example, there are difficult questions about the limits of liberty, paternalistic intervention, and the enforcement of law that are being postponed here. Agents often make unwise or criminal choices that do great harm to themselves or others. Such cases raise both distributive and corrective issues. The habilitation framework is clearly relevant to the distributive issues. And as noted especially in Chapter 9, there is a rebuttable presumption in favor of correcting the damage to health, as a matter of basic justice, for both perpetrators and victims. But in these cases the distributive and corrective issues are intertwined, and there is no claim here that the habilitation framework is by itself adequate for addressing all matters of distributive justice when they are intertwined with corrective ones. Similarly, the damage inflicted by criminal penalties has been treated only in passing, since those are also intertwined with matters of corrective justice. Habilitation into healthy agency is obviously relevant to the choice and application of criminal penalties, but not to the central arguments here.

Voluntary assumption of risk. Additionally, there are two further sets of corrective cases in which the habilitation framework obviously has both relevance and influence, even though I say little about them here. One involves cases in which damage to trait-health occurs as an unintended result of perfectly ordinary, non-culpable activity. There are hazards involved in occupations that are socially necessary, or not necessary but perfectly licit. Police work, for example, or travel. There are hazards involved in pregnancy and childbirth, and disadvantages (sometimes a lifetime of disadvantages) produced by parenthood. Those are clearly cases in which "correction" is habilitation or rehabilitation, and about which normative theories of justice may differ.

Voluntary assumption of damage. The other set of cases involves those in which robustly healthy agents knowingly and voluntarily enter into a way of life that leads away from sustaining their trait-health toward some vision of individual or social perfection which systematically undermines it. Examples include forms of life (religious, intellectual, artistic, athletic, war-fighting) which involve significant, long-term health compromises. Such cases are especially problematic for a eudaimonistic account of health, since in one sense they continue to move forward along the health scale toward its vanishing point of perfection, but in another sense they move backward, by undermining or weakening underlying levels of health. I leave that interesting puzzle for a later time also.

2. Comprehensiveness and Representativeness

Given the exclusions mentioned, are there harmful disadvantages that would necessarily be left untouched by building a theory of justice under the habilitation framework, using the health scale and target of robustly healthy agency proposed here? Reasons for thinking that the answer is no have already been given in previous chapters. But in what follows, a range of cases that might be offered as counterexamples to earlier arguments on this question will be considered.

In each of these cases the reply to these purported counterexamples will take the same form: first, by noting that an effective counterexample will have to offer a case in which something other than health appears to be the distributive issue for justice, and then by arguing that in each case our concern about this proposed counterexample rises or falls in direct relation to its consequences for health, and specifically for robustly healthy agency. If that is so, then health remains the appropriate representative good, and robustly healthy agency remains the appropriate target, in a comprehensive range of cases.

2.1. *Luxuries*

Affluent societies face decisions about distributing resources to the fine arts, higher education, museums, historical sites, national parks, entertainment, recreational facilities, and other things that do not appear to be health-related. So the question is whether the habilitation framework will address those matters at all, and if so, whether it is plausible to think it will address them adequately.

The answer appears to be yes on both counts. As noted in Chapter 3, healthy agency—particularly its psychological factors—may necessarily depend not only on a basic sense of security, trust, confidence, and love for and from others but also on the availability of at least some forms of elevated or transcendent experience. And it is uncontroversial that health is at least nourished by experience that involves admiration, awe, aspiration, adventure, excitement, enthusiasm, delight, engrossing activity, carefree rest, and relaxation. The range of things that has provided such transcendent experience for people is as varied as cathedrals and comedy clubs, tragedies and satyr plays, philosophical conversations and gladiatorial games, the metaphysical poetry of John Donne and the doggerel of the music hall, worshiping a god and watching a soap opera.

Some forms of transcendent or elevated experience are available to people only in a social environment that makes them available. And in large, diverse societies, people's tastes and interests are typically divergent enough that pursuing a public policy goal of robustly healthy agency will require the government to monitor these "luxurious" environmental determinants of health in two ways: by making sure that there is sufficient variety and quantity of such things to provide the necessary health benefits for the entire (relevant) population, and by limiting the variety and quantity of such things insofar as they are detrimental to health.

Much of this (religion, the arts in their avant-garde mode, entertainment in its pop-culture mode, commercially profitable forms of entertainment) may not need redistributive government subsidies, though some of it may need coercive government restraints (chat rooms and e-mail lists devoted to making child pornography; radically militant and revolutionary forms of religious fundamentalism).

It is hard to predict how tethering all of these decisions to health policy would play out in practice. But it is clear enough that they would all be firmly on the habilitative agenda. Also on that agenda would be some limits to what government could reasonably be expected to provide or to involve itself in regulating. And it is plausible to think that normative theories will be able to find those limits somewhere on the health scale in the band that represents robustly healthy agency.

2.2. *Deficits and disabilities*

Using robustly healthy agency (or good health at any level) as the target for distributive justice and public policy will obviously mean that in many cases we will fail to hit the target. Accidents, injuries, diseases, and disasters will intervene to deflect our best efforts in many cases. And age gradually disables us all. A rational goal with respect to that target, then, will be to do the best we can to hit it, understanding that for many people, something less than robustly healthy agency will be the result. This does not mean, however, that they will be left out of distributions once they reach the point where further habilitative progress is impossible.

Implicit in the habilitation framework is a set of ordered preferences for better over lesser forms of health and healthy agency, which includes preferences for greater strength, stability, and range for any given level of health achieved. The social structures necessary to achieve such health throughout the life span, for overlapping generations of citizens, will guarantee the existence of the social structures necessary to sustain (under favorable conditions) whatever level of health is achieved—or at any rate guarantee the existence of social structures whose goal is that pursuit. There are some difficult remainders, but they are no more difficult under this habilitative framework for justice than they are in more conventional ones.

Consider the problem of "what to do with" permanently and severely disabled people. If their agency itself is not impaired but only limited by social or environmental factors, the remedy implicit in the habilitation framework is obvious: make the accommodations necessary to give their agency adequate scope—that is, a scope adequate to provide a reasonable range of choices for an active, productive, full life in a given environment. This habilitative response is directed at the social sources of their disability and is tied to minimizing further habilitative burdens on everyone, including the disabled.

If, however, their agency itself is impaired, independent of social or environmental factors, the appropriate habilitative response is directed at the individual's physical or psychological abilities themselves. If the individual's agency is reparable, then the problem is a rehabilitative one. If not, then the problem is essentially a holding operation—making arrangements that allow whatever agent-activity is possible and good for sustaining the level of health that has been achieved. Again, this habilitative response is tied to minimizing the habilitative burdens on everyone, including the disabled.

In all these cases there are two branching public policy concerns: one is sustaining or improving the level of health the disabled person has achieved; the other is sustaining or improving the level of health achieved by those who will directly or indirectly support the disabled person. These are familiar problems in the discussions of disability and justice, and they are likely to play out in familiar ways under the habilitation framework.

2.3. *When enough health is not enough*

There is no guarantee that robustly healthy agents will be especially satisfied with their lives, especially convivial, especially cooperative, or especially lovable even to their mothers. Suppose they want more wealth, or social recognition, or leisure at public expense? Suppose they don't want merely a good life, but rather the best life they can imagine? Suppose they want a higher level of robust health than is currently the goal of public health policy? Suppose they want optimal health?

These questions are also well within the bounds marked out by the habilitation framework. Robustly healthy agents who don't want more health (or wealth, or whatever is the indexical good), but just want—well—*more* present a familiar set of problems for any theory of justice. And it is reasonable to think that the habilitation framework has the resources to confront them as well, or better, than standard theories taken on their own.

Relative deprivation and healthy levels of resentment and envy. With apologies for brusqueness, consider: problems that come from *healthy* levels of resentment or envy can either be deflected, ignored, or confronted with some version of "Get over it." Those seem to be the options at work in plausible normative theories of justice, and the habilitation framework is neutral between them. Recommending therapy, counseling, reeducation, or special tenderness would imply that we think we are dealing with a deficiency in health which, by hypothesis, we are not.

Health and perfectionism. Problems that come from a desire to achieve the best form of life, where that goes well beyond robustly healthy agency, deserve a more respectful response. But we should note that such desires are drawn not from a conception of basic justice under the general concept of it used here, but rather from a conception of a good life that goes beyond considerations of basic justice. Dealing with the perfectionism that arises from such desires will raise problems for any theory of justice, and any political polity. Basic justice will presumably take priority, and the question will be whether satisfying these additional desires on the part of some people is compatible with it.

The habilitation framework (when it is embedded in a normative theory) will not prejudice the answers that any of the plausible normative theories might give. It will simply ask whether social or political action to encourage or limit perfectionism is necessary, permissible, or useful for meeting the habilitative goals of basic justice, and that goal is common to full-fledged theories of justice. If not, then some version of "Get it yourself" seems appropriate.

If, however, it turns out to be necessary, permissible, or useful to raise the goal from robust health to optimal health, normative theories will run into two familiar problems: one is that the social resources for making such a goal realistic have to be available, either through government programs or through generally accessible private ones. (This assumes social resources will be necessary. It may well be that robustly healthy agents can mostly be left to their own devices in this respect, given the relevant civil liberties.) And the other problem is the extent to which the demand for optimal health will again entangle public policy in disputes between incompatible conceptions of the good. This might be harmless, but it might also be insupportable. Either way, the habilitation framework can address the relevant questions.

If, however, the problems posed by these dissatisfied individuals are essentially challenges to a given political polity itself, we will need to know whether they are problems about a specific instance of that type of polity or more fundamental philosophical problems with the type of polity itself. Either way, these are the sorts of meta-questions any philosophical theory confronts. The habilitation framework confronts them as well.

2.4. *Discrimination and disrespect*

Suppose we have put in place the social structures to create and sustain robustly healthy agents. But suppose that some citizens are subjected to the contempt of others, or disparagement and disrespect, or outright discrimination. Isn't that an injustice that will by definition lie outside the habilitation framework?

The answer is no. Such injustices will *not* lie outside the habilitation framework if they are obstacles to the project of achieving or sustaining robustly healthy agency. They will lie outside the framework only if they are harmless to that project. Mill's famous harm principle, and distinctions between harm and offense based on it, represent a comparable approach to these problems. Surely the potential for discrimination and disrespect to have a withering effect on health and healthy agency is central to an account of *how* they can be more than merely offensive, and how they can be harmful in a way that basic justice cannot ignore.

We regularly give exactly such an account with respect to misogyny, racism, and contempt for the disabled. They take a tragic toll on people's lives when they are systemic, or so widely practiced that they are unavoidable for people on the receiving end, or when the only way of avoiding them is to live a sheltered, limited life. Yet if they do not have even a modest effect on health, even for children and others who are not yet robustly healthy, then it is plausible to think that they are harmless. (This is why ridicule directed against a socioeconomically privileged and dominant group of people is often treated as harmless—or at any rate less harmful than such contemptuous stereotyping of disadvantaged groups.) All of this is standard fare for theories of basic justice. The habilitation framework provides a path to handle such questions within a normative theory, without prejudging the issue.

10

Conclusion and Extrication

Introductions are intended to be disarming in addition to entangling both author and reader in a mutual enterprise. By contrast, what follows is intended solely to disentangle and disengage. Being disarming is no part of the plan.

Intentions often misfire, of course. Introductions may arm a reader to the teeth. Extrications may perversely free the author but deepen the entanglement for everyone else. We will see.

1. Health, Individual Liberty, and Social Stability: A Fantasy

Freedom for the exercise of active, effective agency is built into the habilitation framework from the outset. Self-habilitation is a necessary component of habilitation, and it requires active, effective agency. When such agency is directed toward generating, sustaining, and improving health, the motivation for a wide range of individual freedom for one's agency will be persistent and strong.

For basically healthy agents, however, this motivation will be limited and otherwise integrated into all their habilitative tasks. Recall that people face at least three such tasks, which take different forms throughout their lives: getting the habilitation sufficient for their own welfare, through their own efforts and the efforts of others; helping to habilitate others to the extent necessary for them, and for themselves; and helping to habilitate the physical and social environment where necessary for themselves and others. All those habilitative tasks aim at, and ultimately require, a genuinely hospitable physical and social environment, as does healthy agency itself. So the motivation for generating, sustaining, and improving a hospitable environment, characterized in part by a sufficient population of other basically healthy agents, will also be persistent and strong.

This has the effect of motivating a political liberty principle framed in terms of habilitation. Basic good health will be characterized by the motivation toward forms of individual freedom that are non-self-destructive and non-self-defeating, both at the individual level and the social level, while at the same time being as expansive as possible for the individual. (This is not a distributive rule—an equal liberty principle—but it certainly leans in that direction within the population of basically healthy individuals.)

The fantasy is that basic good health and healthy agency, when sufficiently widespread throughout a population, will itself have the consequence of strengthening and stabilizing a hospitable social environment characterized by extensive individual liberty for the whole population. And it is also part of the fantasy that such a social environment will be characterized by greatly reduced violence and coercion, moving those things first toward conflicts that are resolved by cooperation, and then ultimately away from persistent conflict and cooperation problems toward mere coordination problems.

Traffic rules illustrate the possibilities. Driving on the wrong side of the road in heavy traffic (absent emergencies) is so deeply stupid that it rarely even causes coordination problems, let alone cooperation problems or conflict. For the most part, it is effectively coordinated simply by an agreed-upon convention, with agreed-upon exceptions. Violating the convention is a sign of dementia, intoxication, wanton recklessness, or confusion. Speeding, however, currently requires some persistent enforcement, since for many people cooperation with speed limits quickly degrades without it. And some annoying but perfectly legal lane-changing behavior is managed by size and aggression in situations that are effectively contests or conflicts. The right-of-way there goes to the biggest vehicles and most aggressive drivers. A similar variety of problems plagues many sorts of social interactions.

The fantasy, then, is that the motivation of healthy agents will be strongly cooperative to begin with, which will reduce conflict and increase the extent to which cooperation problems become at most coordination problems, with modest arrangements for enforcement. But healthy agents will also be strongly oriented toward individual freedom. They will restrict it only to the extent necessary for non-self-destructive and non-self-defeating forms of habilitation—the peaceable kingdom of the healthy.

This is only a fantasy, of course. I confess it is one I cherish, and it is no doubt part of my motivation for pursuing this project. But I am not so fond of it that I fail to see that what passes for basic good health is often an easily shattered appearance. And even when it is a reality, it is no guarantee of a tranquil, cooperative existence among the healthy.

2. Approximations to Health

Basic good health is a very demanding target. Most people who appear to have it actually have only an approximation of it—and one that is a close approximation only in a limited range of environments. If they are lucky they can manage to function competently at quite a distance from robustly healthy agency, and in lucky social circumstances, the whole society can remain stable with widely varying approximations to healthy agency throughout the population.

But we are often unlucky, and bad luck is often catastrophic and irreversible. What is the foreseeable prospect that we can eliminate catastrophic human endowments, disease, injury, traumatic social experience? What is the prospect that we can eliminate catastrophic events in the physical environment that have catastrophic effects on human health? What is the prospect that we can eliminate the possibility of choosing, or submitting to, or being subjected to charismatic but deeply pathological leaders? Or eliminate the possibility of the widespread development of pathologically fixed attachments, or pathologically self-destructive (but otherwise charming and reliably competent) personalities in a given population? Nil, in all those cases.

For the foreseeable future, the reality is that most human individuals will fall short of basic good health, and many will fall far short of it. Moreover, it looks as though some societies will be chronically short of sufficiency in either the raw number or the distribution of basically healthy agents—in families, neighborhoods, schools, businesses, and communities; locally, nationally, globally. These shortfalls will slow or in some cases reverse progress toward basic good health for individuals and populations. Such chronic shortfalls will be self-sustaining insofar as they generate a constant supply of pathological human agents and only approximately healthy ones locked into intractable, self-destructive, and self-defeating conflicts in every level of the social environment.

None of this troubles my confidence in this project. It still seems clear that basic good health is among the things that are good for everyone and that progress toward it is better than stasis or a decline away from it, other things being equal. And it still seems clear that progress toward basic justice is most reliable when its norms are motivated by healthy agency itself, perhaps reinforced by one of the competing normative theories consistent with both individual health and basic justice. So other things equal, the more widespread basic good health is throughout the population, the better off everyone will be, at least in terms of reliably creating and reliably sustaining the sorts of environments that are basically just and hospitable.

3. Pseudo-problems and Elusive Targets: Sensible Replies to the Foole

Still, basic good health and robustly healthy agency are elusive and mostly aspirational targets. It doesn't take much to generate troublesome thoughts about their troublesome aspects. Usually these are nighttime doubts raised only by one's inner

Foole. Most of them are uninteresting, but some of them deserve a sensible public Reply.

Foole: Is it necessarily better *for me* if *you* make progress toward basic good health? Is it necessarily better *for all of us* if more and more people make progress toward basic good health? I ask, because if I have to choose between a robustly healthy enemy and one whose health is unstable or weak, I think I would want to choose the weak one. And that goes for populations as well. I'd rather keep all my enemies weak, wouldn't I?

Reply. Why do you think that a robustly healthy agent would be your enemy? An adversary, possibly. Or a competitor. But such an agent would be every bit as much aware of habilitative necessities as you are, and every bit as much committed to cooperation toward accomplishing habilitative tasks. And isn't progress toward robustly healthy agency necessarily progress toward such habilitative commitments? Why wouldn't you want your social world full of people making such progress, if you can get it? Some of them still might oppose you on particular issues you hold dear, but they would be worthy opponents, worthy adversaries, worthy competitors in part to the extent that they approximate robustly healthy agency. There is more to worthiness than that, of course, which is why we need more than basic justice—and perhaps more than basically good health. But surely progress toward the basic kind is nothing to fear.

Foole: I'm not so sure. In the absence of the "more" that you so casually now introduce, it seems to me there's a lot to fear. This something "more" involved in worthiness presumably comes from regions of justice and morality that you have systematically avoided throughout this discussion. And without more in the way of morality and justice than basic good health itself motivates, some robustly healthy agents might well be my enemies—and much more formidable enemies than less healthy ones.

Reply: Is that because you yourself are less than a robustly healthy Foole, and you think your enmity against those who are healthy would come from your own lack of it? That is, are you the one who fails to see habilitative necessities, or to cooperate with habilitative tasks? If so, there is no answer to that, other than what has been given throughout the book.

Or is your reason rather that you think conflict—perhaps even war—among robustly healthy agents is inevitable? If so, we can agree on that.

What we evidently can't agree on is any attempt to make your robustly healthy enemies less healthy than they are, and to keep the rest of your enemies from making progress toward basic good health. After all, if we have to have conflicts, or even wars, we still want them to end in the sort of peace that can be preserved—the sort that is stable and resistant to regression back toward war; the sort that leaves us with at least the possibility of a genuinely hospitable physical and social environment. It would take a very long book to demonstrate that the likelihood of getting that sort of end to conflict is not improved when people on both sides of the conflict either exhibit or are making progress toward basic good health.

Foole: [After an unconvinced silence.] There is another question about health as the target that is worrisome. Isn't basic good health—especially in its psychological dimension—ultimately like happiness, in that it is better pursued indirectly rather than directly? Wouldn't we be better off going after other things that have basic good health as a by-product? Like liberty, education, or economic resources?

Reply: That indirect route is the one we have been taking for millennia. The record has been disappointing. Improvements in individual health and population health often do occur as by-products—or certainly are correlated with improvements in socioeconomic status, educational achievement, and the elimination of discrimination and oppression. But it is disappointing to see how often treating health as a by-product leads to misplaced efforts at economic or social development, tracking the effects on health, if at all, with misguided measures such as simple longevity or subjective life satisfaction. And it is even more disappointing to see how often health gets shoved out of the picture almost entirely in the focus on "other things."

Foole: How can it be otherwise, if you insist on making duties out of habilitative necessities. Couldn't the ancient Greek and Roman philosophers have made something like the following argument? Can you avoid the conclusion?

1. Mining is an economic necessity. It is, of course, damaging to the health of the miners, but that is the price of economic progress. So we need to arrange to get people to work in the mines despite the damage it does to their health.
2. We will ask for citizen volunteers. If we do not get such volunteers in sufficient numbers, we will offer incentives. And if those incentives are insufficient, we will manage to restrict the options of potential miners to make mining the most attractive one available.
3. If those forms of more or less voluntary cooperation also fail, or threaten to fail, we will conscript miners, just as we conscript soldiers. And if conscription for mining is politically impossible to sustain within society, we will go outside, to noncitizens, and go through the same process: volunteers, incentivized volunteers, limited-option volunteers, conscripts.
4. In some circumstances, conscripts working in the mines will have to be slaves. And the world we live in now is one such circumstance.

Let's hear your answer.

Reply: Such arguments are incompatible with the motivations of even approximately healthy agency in favorable circumstances. Unfortunately, those arguments are regularly compatible with the way those motivations get translated into practice. But that is no reason for giving up on the pursuit of robustly healthy agency. Instead, it is a powerful reason for thinking that basic good health will ultimately be an obstacle to the forms of self-deception, distorted forms of consciousness, and rationalizations that sustain slavery and other practices which systematically, and coercively, degrade the health of some human beings for the benefit of others. It will not, by itself, be an effective barrier. And it is not, by itself, a distributive principle. That is, we still need a normative theory of basic justice to go with the habilitation framework and its emphasis on health and healthy agency. But when basic good health is widely distributed throughout the population, *and supported by an egalitarian normative principle with respect to the distribution of health*, it will be a powerful barrier against basic injustice.

Consider slavery. Unless we are prepared to say that all the political philosophers and other writers in ancient Greece and Rome lacked even a close approximation to robustly healthy agency, we will have to acknowledge that it is compatible with a form of consciousness that screens out *even the question* of the justice of the institution of slavery. We know that many questions about slavery were raised in discussions of justice. But these were questions about the acquisition, status, use, punishment, manumission, and general treatment of slaves. They did not, as far as we know, reach the question of the justice of the institution of slavery itself.[1]

---

[1] For the Greeks, consider Plato's *Laws*, in which the just treatment of slaves is discussed at length; and of course Aristotle, who gives voice to the view that some people are "natural" slaves. For the Romans, see Bradley, *Slaves and Masters in the Roman Empire* (1987), throughout, but especially at p. 35, in reference to Tacitus. Julia Annas, however, in *Intelligent Virtue* (2011, 59–65), argues that "The Roman Stoics . . . disagree with Aristotle [about the naturalness of slavery]. Virtuous people, they hold, belong to the universal community of rational beings, and from this viewpoint can realize that slavery has no natural or ethical basis . . . [but is] completely conventional." We then of course have to explain the lack of opposition, in their texts, to the institution itself, as opposed to various ways of abusing slaves.

But historically, slavery was an accepted practice worldwide for many millennia, both in preliterate and literate societies, and the conscious, deliberate, and ruthless lack of mutual recognition involved in it make it a special problem. See Orlando Patterson, *Slavery and Social Death* (1992), which opens with this statement:

> There is nothing notably peculiar about the institution of slavery. It has existed from before the dawn of human history right down to the 20th century, in the most primitive of human societies and in the most civilized. There is no region on earth that has not at some time harbored the institution. Probably there is no group of people whose ancestors were not at one time slaves or slaveholders. Why then the commonplace that slavery is 'the peculiar institution'? It is hard to say, but perhaps the reason lies in the tendency to eschew what seems too paradoxical. Slavery was not only ubiquitous but turns out to have thrived most in precisely those areas and periods of the world where our conventional wisdom would lead us to expect it least. It was formally established in all the great early centers of human civilization and, far from declining, actually increased in significance with the growth of all the epochs and cultures that modern Western peoples consider watersheds in their historical development. Ancient Greece and Rome were not simply slaveholding societies; they were what Sir Moses Finley calls 'genuine' slave societies, in that slavery was very solidly the base of their socioeconomic structures. (vii)

It appears that the source of this was a combination of their approximation to healthy agency combined with a settled distributive principle, or tradition, or form of consciousness which did not allow them to raise the question. Perhaps they thought some people deserved to be slaves, or were natural slaves, or were fated to be slaves. And perhaps some of them thought that people who were enslaved for whatever reason would thereby be outside the bounds of the moral community.

Some of this was evidently true even for the Stoics. And that is alternately a bitter disappointment and a troubling puzzle. The ancient Stoics deliberately constructed an account of virtue that was inclusive and universal. Virtue, for them, was not just the highest good; it was the only good, and it was equally accessible to emperors and slaves, foreigners and citizens, men and women. Moreover, their account of virtue was closely linked to their account of human health, and in particular the full development of rational agency, the perfection of which they identified with virtue. Rational agency, they held, was extraordinarily difficult to perfect and required both strenuous efforts by the agents themselves and considerable help from others. But it was possible to make progress, by diligent effort. And they evidently thought many people did make such progress, whether they were slaves or emperors. Some Stoics had a good deal to say about the unjust treatment of slaves; Seneca is an example. But again, those discussions were about how the institution of slavery should be arranged, *in order to be just.* They apparently never reached the question of the injustice of the institution itself.

This is difficult to explain in a fully satisfactory way, especially for the Stoics. They were not setting out to explicate the moral concerns of their local communities, granting their own communities some sort of peremptory validity. They were able, in many other cases, to extricate themselves from conventional modes of thought. And if they admitted women and slaves to their schools, as they did, and if some of them addressed the question of the equality of women with a seriousness that was unusual for the time, why were they so silent about slavery? It is a puzzle.

Foole: You are sliding off my question. I am suggesting that the habilitation framework itself is complicit, in the following way—and I will use your own words against you: framing questions of basic justice in terms of habilitation invites the focus on eudaimonistic health, basic good health, and robustly healthy agency. A

He goes on to document this not only in 460 pages of text and notes but also in Appendix B, which charts mostly preliterate slaveholding societies in the Murdock World Sample, and in Appendix C, which charts large-scale slave systems in literate societies around the world—ancient, medieval, Renaissance, and modern.

part of that focus is an entanglement with habilitative necessities, including the necessity of a genuinely hospitable physical and social environment. The motivational structure and behavioral dispositions of healthy agents will be oriented strongly toward securing things that are habilitative necessities, and oriented strongly toward opposing things that make securing those necessities impossible or improbable or even difficult. The circumstances of habilitation include behavioral tendencies toward strong attachments and forms of radiating benevolence that give the highest priority to the self and its strongest attachments. Thus the table is set for the following kind of false consciousness, in the form of a set of largely implicit fixed beliefs:

1. Mining is a habilitative necessity in this environment. It is a self-destructive choice that no rational agent would make voluntarily. (It differs in this regard from serving in combat, or putting one's life at risk in childbearing. Both of those are paths to honor and glory. They are admired for their own sake, because they express virtue and courage and are not merely means to an inferior, albeit necessary, economic end.)
2. So mining will have to be made a matter of enforceable duty, making it effectively a matter of conscription in many cases.
3. But habilitative necessities dictate that those conscripted be ones that the society can afford to lose, as well as ones who are well-suited for the work. Ultimately, that means slaves.

Can't there be a kernel of honesty in this?

Reply: Yes—in the way that any argument riddled with mistakes can still be honest. And we should remember that physical and social environments can be very harsh, and the line between hospitable ones and unsurvivable ones can be very thin. Where our survival is threatened persistently, we are tempted to defend ourselves first and ask questions about mistakes in our arguments about justice later.

But there is also a grave, subliminal temptation to be dishonest, or blind. Not too long ago by historical standards, we heard arguments about the economic necessity of slavery and the social, political, economic, psychological, and even medical necessity for the subordination of women. Often these things receive only subdued or isolated and ineffective comment for lengthy periods.

Still, my point was that this does not indicate a lack of approximate good health, or approximately healthy agency. Rather, it may indicate that the approximation is flawed in a particularly damaging way. The remedy for that is complex and may involve simply trading one form of approximation for another less damaging one. Even so, that change can be significant.

In cases of moral blindness, for example, one of the things we need is a closer approximation to robustly healthy agency in three particular respects: (1) One of these is in the extent to which the agent possesses the elements of practical reasoning which match up directly with elements of natural justice. Those elements include commitments to impartiality, consistency, and principled conduct justifiable by reasoning that does not rely upon an esoteric epistemology available only to people with certain religious, ethnic, or political identities. (2) Another is the extent to which agents tether deliberation and choice (a) to an experimental method that is vigilant about searching for, and adjusting decisions to reflect, evidence that invalidates the choice; (b) to an appreciation of the strategic nature of the conduct involved, and the limitations of human knowledge generally; and (c) to the dangers of fixed beliefs that are insensitive to evidence. (3) The third is the extent to which agents remain capable of mutual recognition, mutual respect, mutual benevolence, and reciprocity.

Of course, robustly healthy agency doesn't guarantee the implementation of basic justice under any particular distributive principle. It only motivates implementing it under some reasonable distributive principle. And in some of its approximations, the motivation intrinsic to healthy agency can apparently support some disgusting distributive principles. But in our lifetimes, we have seen the way in which consciousness of the injustice of antisemitism, racism, and many forms of sexism is being raised at least in large part by improving healthy agency. It may be that healthy agency itself is never sufficient for such tasks. But it is plausible to think that it is necessary. Any progress against such injustices is likely to be unstable and local if it cannot be made in these terms, even if it often has to be sold, politically, in other ways.

Foole: Still unconvincing. And there is a closely related part of the same problem. It is that some approximately healthy agents remain motivated to move toward social isolation. To some extent that motivation is a product of the different degrees of solidarity that develop among people depending on the intimacy, frequency, and rewardingness of their relationships. And to some extent the motivation is a product of danger or threat of danger from others. In either case, social groups, large and small, may become closed to others. Membership becomes tightly defined and borders tightly controlled. Habilitative duties to nonmembers are sharply limited. Allegiances to large, diverse social groups are replaced by allegiances to smaller, less diverse groups—perhaps those with a shared ethnic or religious identity. And the group itself may have isolating internal partitions: the division of labor may harden into a class system or be closed altogether into a caste system. Communication within or between groups may become difficult. And this may have consequences for individuals, who then may isolate themselves further by refusing to have nothing more than minimal dealings with those outside their families, or religious or ethnic or political groups. In extreme cases, individuals may avoid even those contacts.

We cannot write this off entirely as pathology—at least in its beginnings. And it cannot always be put down to a flawed normative theory of justice. To repeat: a significant part of it can develop from the interaction between approximately healthy agents living in harsh or threatening environments.

The sequence can go something like this. When it is especially difficult to meet habilitative necessities, we tend to simplify the necessary tasks, find solutions that work reliably and efficiently, and stay with them. One important way we can achieve this is by living and working among the people with whom we have the strongest solidarity, based on mutual respect, trust, and genuinely reciprocal relationships. Then when the physical or social environment is not only difficult but dangerous and threatening, we must also spend a good deal of time defending ourselves. In that case we may begin to isolate ourselves out of a sense that it is necessary for self-defense, and then begin to think that isolation might be necessary or at least expedient for all our habilitative tasks even in the absence of imminent dangers.

When such thoughts become fixed beliefs, perhaps reinforced by the religious or political culture, what started as an interaction between approximately healthy agents in an especially harsh environment soon begins to degrade such agency in familiar ways. And it can be difficult for people to make their way out of a degenerative, self-destructive and self-defeating cycle characterized by increasingly desperate attempts to isolate themselves in ways that take them farther and farther from the norms of basic justice.

Reply: Habilitation into robustly healthy agency is fortunately a persistent project. But unless it is also characterized by persistent motivation to increase the range of environments in which people are reliably competent to function, healthy agency by itself may not be adequate to break this sort of degenerative cycle. People within progressively more isolated social environments may not only lose the competence to function in other environments but also the competence to function in their own environment if it (re)engages with others.

In a world that is truly interdependent, however, we can rely on closer and closer approximations to robustly healthy agency to keep us aware of that interdependence and its effect on habilitative tasks. That will keep us at least ambivalent about our isolationist tendencies, and presumably supportive of a conception of robustly healthy agency that is competent to function reliably in a wide range of environments. We may not ourselves be able to achieve this widely competent form of agency, but we will come to see that as a limitation in ourselves. And we will be motivated toward mutual recognition, respect, reciprocity, and the universal implementation of the norms of basic justice.

Consider human rights. Rights to the things that are habilitative necessities, especially the things necessary for basic good health, will be clearly and ubiquitously in focus. But they will be most naturally understood as correlatives to human duties, because it is duties that seem to emerge most directly from the attempt to represent habilitative necessities as normative requirements.

These normative requirements will be *human* duties and their correlative rights will be *human* rights, insofar as habilitative necessities arise for all humans. But it is important to notice that the details will vary according to the habilitative possibilities available within a given environment. We cannot have duties of basic justice to provide things for ourselves and others that are physically or socially impossible to produce. (Example: it may not be possible in some societies to provide, by a date certain, the advantages of modern medicine or democratic political organization.) And the details will vary further according to the habilitative possibilities available for particular individuals given their particular physical and psychological endowments, development, and health. (We might have duties to prohibit deracinated individuals from registering to vote.)

This account of human rights embeds them firmly in our most fundamental justice-connected project as human beings—habilitation—and defines their content and priority by reference to actual habilitative necessities and possibilities. Sometimes, human rights are presented politically as if they were self-evident absolutes, applicable across cultures without modifications or priorities based on the physical and social circumstances involved. That may be inspiring rhetoric at a religious level, or for human rights activists, but when it is embedded in a normative theory of justice, it is problematic. At least it is problematic if it doesn't give appropriate weight to local difficulties in implementing such rights. (This takes us back to something that should have been mentioned earlier: Hart's critique of the lexical priority of an equal liberty principle.)

The other reason this result is welcome is that it addresses the perpetrators of injustice directly, by reminding them first of the duties they have to others and linking those duties to the necessities for basic good health. Habilitation is a goal everyone can understand immediately, and the importance of health to habilitation is a simple, convincing inference to make.

It is not hard to identify, in a given environment, the most fundamental habilitative necessities, possibilities, and priorities for basic good health. This is something any approximately competent rational agent can understand. Reminding approximately healthy despots of their duties with respect to their own and others' health (and by implication, the rights of others to good health) is quite possibly a better strategic move than starting with lists of human rights that appear to come out of nowhere—or worse, appear to come out of the meddlesome moralizing of foreign governments or alien religions. The conversation will come around to correlative human rights soon enough.

Foole: This is a result that may not be entirely welcome for normative theories that make rights the fundamental moral category. They might want to insist that human rights come from a source independent of habilitative necessities—that they come instead from a special dignity possessed by each human being. And they might want to insist that such human rights are importantly invariant across cultures and across the diversity of individual human endowments, development, and health—at least as enforceable prohibitions of the worst forms of injustice against the personhood of each individual.

Reply: Invoking human dignity as a ground for human rights is alternately inspiring and alienating. Inspiring because it leads us to reflect on what it is that might be infinitely precious and unique to each human being: personhood, as we say, or perhaps the reflective, intentional self-consciousness of each person. But alienating as well, since it is hard to avoid asking, under one's breath, dignity in what respect? And compared to whom? Rational agency of the form that leads to genocidal wars, or even petty malice, is not dignified. And even if that will not do—even if each person is uniquely and infinitely precious in a sense that is not sullied by his or her actual thoughts, and actual behavior, the path from that unique value to the claim of inalienable rights is obscure. There is a gap between unique value and unique rights. As for dignity in a less metaphysical sense, arguing from our subjective appreciation of ourselves, it is undoubtedly true that most of us are psychologically attached to ourselves and to those who are dear to our own dear selves. And perhaps some of us find human beings generally endearing. But admiring ourselves doesn't make us admirable. And wanting to believe that human beings have some kind of infinite, special dignity doesn't make it a fact that we do have it—not to mention that human history is not exactly replete with it (present company excepted, of course).

An old-fashioned approach may be better. Begin with the recognition that despite the fact that human beings have certain charming prosocial propensities, we are pretty scary creatures and in many ways disgusting ones. Without internalized norms of justice we regularly wind up behaving atrociously to each other and everything else, usually while continuing to wallow in self-love. So it seems that the hunt for human dignity as a *premise* for justice has turned things upside down. The premise instead should be that what makes justice both possible and necessary is that without it, we have no special dignity at all—just a thin, watchful form of cooperative social behavior concealing a ferocious, feral psychology.

And from that premise the theory of justice that comes most immediately to mind is one ultimately based on duties and not on rights—duties that originate in the moral necessity, for each of us, of turning our dear, feral selves into something more admirable and dignified, and capable of living cooperatively and even affectionately with each other. There is no special dignity-conferring property that we need to find in order to go down this path toward the justification of duties. Political philosophy got along in this way long before the invention of rights originating in the glories of human nature.

Duty-based theories of justice can be very powerful and need not be repressive, illiberal, or exclusionary. There are duties of benevolence, care, and cooperation as well as mutual advantage; duties of intervention as well as duties of self-restraint. All of them can be understood as generating correlative rights. And all of them can be grounded in habilitative necessities.

The habilitation framework is certainly in principle open to a normative theory that takes rights and human dignity as more fundamental than duties. It is not open, however, to ignoring the diversity of habilitative necessities and possibilities across physical and social environments, and across individuals.

That is, I think, likely to be an advantage for people working out normative accounts of global justice. Part of that process must surely be the recognition of diversity. And the process must also be sensitive to the way in which the rhetoric of human rights often encounters resistance when it appears to pull a list of right claims out of thin air, or out of a contestable normative theory, or out of a particular political tradition. Duties (and correlative rights) based on habilitative necessities, and explicitly defined in terms of the necessities and possibilities of particular physical and social environments are perhaps likely to encounter less resistance (and hypocritical assent) than lists of human rights—especially if those duties are about basic good health of a eudaimonistic sort.

4. Hope rather than Fantasy

All these difficulties and dangers notwithstanding, it is not a fantasy to imagine that if we can ever achieve large populations of people who closely approximate basic good health—and especially healthy agency—throughout a preponderance of influential social environments in the world, we will have done an enormous amount toward making basic justice secure.

We will have created at least some large, stable, and genuinely hospitable social environments in which both basic good health and basic justice are secure internally, absent catastrophic disasters.

We will have created a global social environment in which the extension of such basic good health and basic justice to all other social environments is much more likely than it is now.

And if all that were to happen, the worst forms of injustice that humans do to each other would be much reduced—at least in frequency and extent.

Given the slim chance that there will ever be general agreement on a comprehensive conception of the good or a comprehensive normative theory of justice (let alone compliance with it), this may be the most we can aspire to without definitely going into the land of pure fantasy.

Moreover, by increasing the range of environments in which agents can function competently and reliably, we will have increased the number and variety of navigable paths to a good life for very many people who otherwise would have had very limited prospects.

And it looks as though all of this would make it possible to integrate ordinary notions of happiness into the conception of basic good health, since the causal connection between it and positive emotional and affective states is now fairly clear.

That is sufficiently inspiring for a set of philosophical proposals about a mere framework for building theories of justice—if those proposals are sound, of course. Striving for more inspiration from them, like more happiness, would be self-defeating. Not to mention unseemly.

Acknowledgments

This book began with some promising ideas that I tried unsuccessfully to shrug off onto other people for further work, which led in turn to a succession of equally unsuccessful attempts to write up these ideas much more briefly, and then at significantly greater length than what is found here. The result is a testimony to the patience and persistence of friends, colleagues, students, and editors. It is not a very flattering testimony to my readiness to listen, though I eventually did, mostly.

There is a substantial list of people who deserve special acknowledgment. Since those who helped in the early stages of the project were every bit as influential as those who pored over the nearly final manuscript, a chronological approach to these matters seems in order.

Gestural versions of some of this material were presented in lectures and symposia: at APA symposia in 2003 and 2008 (on Martha Nussbaum's then-forthcoming *Frontiers of Justice*, and Jonathan Wolff and Avner de-Shalit's then-recently-published *Disadvantage*, respectively); in lectures to a conference on positive psychology at the University of Pennsylvania (2003), to the advisory committee of the National Institutes of Health's National Center for Medical Rehabilitation Research (2004), to the graduate department of rehabilitation engineering at the University of Pittsburgh (2004), to a multi-university colloquium in bioethics held at Georgetown University (2007), and in two connected lectures at Virginia Tech in April 2009. I am indebted to participants in all these events for comments that have produced some course corrections in my project, and have improved some of my arguments.

In 2008, my attempt to distill some of these arguments into a single journal article understandably failed to convince the editors and referees. Their extensive and careful comments convinced me that the project was hopelessly sketchy at 10,000 words, and would be no better at double that length. So I began this book in late 2008. Drafts of a manuscript were circulated to participants in a symposium on this and other aspects of my work at the American Philosophical Association's Central Division meetings in February 2010. Most of the speakers commented on the manuscript, either during the symposium or in preparation for it, and all of these comments have prompted improvements. Special thanks for discussion on that occasion go to Elizabeth Fenton, Michael Gettings, Paula Gottlieb, Margaret Graver, Leslie Francis, John Partridge, Anita Silvers, and Peter Vallentyne. The comments delivered by Margaret Graver, with subsequent comments by Anita Silvers, may be found in the *APA Newsletter on Philosophy and Medicine*, Fall 2010.

Beginning in late 2009, Leslie Francis and Jonathan Wolff read subsequent versions of the entire manuscript and offered valuable observations throughout about how it could be clarified or strengthened. In particular, their remarks led me to confront more directly, and I think more convincingly, the worry of many readers that the habilitation framework might be a full-fledged normative theory in disguise. They also prompted me to do something with what had been a very long and leisurely chapter on the circumstances of habilitation. I have no idea whether they will think this final version is responsive, or responsive enough, to their suggestions. So it is not just pro forma to say that they bear no responsibility for my remaining errors and lack of clarity. But they certainly deserve, and have, my gratitude.

Anita Silvers has, over many years, been a persistent and particularly helpful influence, both on the direction of my thinking on justice and on my motivation to get on with this project. I have also had especially fruitful exchanges about specific parts of the manuscript with Asha Bhandary, John Christman, Michael Gettings, Paula Gottlieb, Margaret Graver, John Kekes, Corey Keyes, and Thomas Lawson. Again, I do not mean to imply their agreement with my approach here, or with my arguments.

Partial or full drafts of the manuscript have also been discussed in an interdisciplinary graduate seminar on justice at Hollins University. My thanks go to all the students in the 2009, 2010, and 2011 editions of that seminar, but especially to Deborah Basham, Jessie Coffman, John Heaton, Jeffery Hodges, Jeffery Kennard, Lauren Lehmann, Stewart MacInnis, Elizabeth Mortlock, and Joel Shinofield.

Reginald Tyler, my travel wrangler from 1993 to 2010, made it possible for me to get to out-of-town events during those years, including to many conferences where the ideas in this book were shaped by what I heard, rather than by what was specifically on the program. Reggie's friendship and encouragement, as well as his astute and practical comments on matters of health and agency, were important to the work on this book, and remain important to me personally.

As is evident from this skeletal history, turning these ideas about habilitation, health, and agency into a book has been anything but a solitary enterprise. My editor at Oxford University Press, Peter Ohlin, has been extraordinarily steady and patient, as has been his team of anonymous reviewers. It has been a delight to work with the Press's editorial assistants and production staff as well.

This book is dedicated to Charlotte, my wife of forty-five years. Her support for the project, as well as for everything else I have undertaken over the years, has been so encompassing that a mere dedication is paltry. She is my most astute critic; my most important collaborator on shared projects; and my most supportive, constant, and loving friend. In a fundamental sense, the existence of this book—and my own continued existence—is a gift of love from her.

Bibliography

American Psychiatric Association. *Diagnostic and Statistical Manual of Mental Disorders*, 4th ed. Washington, DC: American Psychiatric Association, 1994.

Anderson, Elizabeth. "What Is the Point of Equality?" *Ethics* 109:2 (1999): 287–337.

———. "Justifying the Capabilities Approach to Justice." In *Measuring Justice: Primary Goods and Capabilities*, edited by Harry Brighouse and Ingrid Robeyns, 81–100. New York: Cambridge University Press, 2010.

Annas, Julia. *The Morality of Happiness*. New York: Oxford University Press, 1993.

———. *Intelligent Virtue*. New York: Oxford University Press, 2011.

Archer, John. *Ethology and Human Development*. Lanham, MD: Rowman and Littlefield, 1992.

Ariely, Dan. *Predictably Irrational: The Hidden Forces That Shape Our Decisions*. New York: Harper, 2008.

Arneson, Richard. "Equality and Equality of Opportunity for Welfare." *Philosophical Studies* 56 (1989): 77–93.

———. "Liberalism, Distributive Subjectivism, and Equal Opportunity for Welfare." *Philosophy and Public Affairs* 19 (1990): 158–94.

Baier, Annette. "The Need for More than Justice." In Annette Baier, *Moral Prejudices*. Cambridge: Cambridge University Press, 1994.

Barry, Brian, and Russell Hardin, eds. *Rational Man and Irrational Society: An Introduction and Source Book*. Beverly Hills: Sage, 1982.

Battin, Margaret P., Leslie P. Francis, Jay A. Jacobson, and Charles B. Smith. *The Patient as Victim and Vector: Ethics and Infectious Disease*. New York: Oxford University Press, 2009.

Becker, Lawrence C. "The Finality of Moral Judgments." *Philosophical Review* 82 (1973a): 364–71.

———. *On Justifying Moral Judgments*. London: Routledge and Kegan Paul, 1973b.

———. *Reciprocity*. London: Routledge and Kegan Paul, 1986.

———. "Community, Dominion, and Membership." *Southern Journal of Philosophy* 30:3 (1992a): 17–43.

———. "Good Lives: Prolegomena." *Social Philosophy and Policy* 9 (1992b): 5–37. Reprinted in *The Good Life and the Human Good*, edited by Ellen Frankel Paul. Cambridge: Cambridge University Press, 1993.

———. *A New Stoicism*. Princeton: Princeton University Press, 1998a.

———. "Stoic Children." In *The Philosopher's Child: Critical Essays in the Western Tradition*, edited by Susan M. Turner and Gareth B. Matthews, 45–61. Rochester, NY: University of Rochester Press, 1998b.

———. "Stoic Emotion." In *Stoicism: Traditions and Transformations*, edited by Jack Zupko and Steven K. Strange, 250–75. New York: Cambridge University Press, 2004.

———. "Reciprocity, Justice, and Disability." *Ethics* 116:1 (October 2005): 9–39.

Berk, Laura E. *Child Development*, 8th ed. Boston: Allyn and Bacon, 2008.

Bickle, John, ed. *The Oxford Handbook of Philosophy and Neuroscience*. New York: Oxford University Press, 2009.

Bok, Sissela. *Common Values*, 2nd ed. Columbia: University of Missouri Press, 2002.

———. "WHO Definition of Health, Rethinking the." In *International Encyclopedia of Public Health*, Vol. 6, edited by Kris Heggenhougen and Stella Quah, 590–97. San Diego: Academic Press, 2008.

Boorse, Christopher. "On the Distinction between Disease and Illness." *Philosophy and Public Affairs* 5:1 (1975): 49–68.

———. "What a Theory of Mental Health Should Be." *Journal of the Theory of Social Behavior* 6:1 (1976): 61–84.

———. "Health as a Theoretical Concept." *Philosophy of Science* 44:4 (1977): 542–73.

———. "A Rebuttal on Health." In *What Is Disease?* edited by J. M. Humber and R. F. Almeder, 1–134. Totowa, NJ: Humana Press, 1997.

Bradley, K. R. *Slaves and Masters in the Roman Empire: A Study in Social Control*. New York: Oxford University Press, 1987.

Brighouse, Harry, and Ingrid Robeyns, eds. *Measuring Justice: Primary Goods and Capabilities*. New York: Cambridge University Press, 2010.

Buchanan, Allen. "Justice and Charity." *Ethics* 97:3 (1987): 558–75.

———. *Justice and Health Care*. New York: Oxford University Press, 2009.

Chodorow, Nancy. *The Reproduction of Mothering*, 1st ed. 1978; updated edition 1999. Berkeley: University of California Press, 1999.

Churchland, Patricia S. *Brain Trust: What Science Tells Us about Morality*. Princeton: Princeton University Press, 2011.

Cicero, Marcus Tulius. *De Finibus.*

Cloninger, C. Robert. *Feeling Good: The Science of Well-Being*. New York: Oxford University Press, 2004.

———. "The Science of Well-Being: An Integrated Approach to Mental Health and Its Disorders." *World Psychiatry* 5 (2006): 71–76.

Cloninger, C. Robert, Ada Zohar, and Kevin M. Cloninger, "Promotion of Well-Being in Person-Centered Mental Health Care." *Focus* 8:2 (2010): 165–78.

Clouser, K. Danner, Charles M. Culver, and Bernard Gert. "Malady." In *What Is Disease?* edited by J. M. Humber and R. F. Almeder, 175–217. Totowa, NJ: Humana Press, 1997.

Coetzee, J. M. *Elizabeth Costello*. New York: Viking, 2003.

Cohen, G. A. "On the Currency of Egalitarian Justice." *Ethics* 99 (1989): 906–44.

———. "Equality of What? On Welfare, Goods and Capabilities." In *Quality of Life*, edited by Amartya Sen and Martha Nussbaum. Oxford: Clarendon Press, 1993.

———. *Rescuing Justice and Equality*. Cambridge, MA: Harvard University Press, 2008.

———. *Why Not Socialism?* Princeton: Princeton University Press, 2009.

Comin, Flavio. "Measuring Capabilities." In *The Capability Approach: Concepts, Measures, and Applications*, edited by Flavio Comin, Mozaffar Qizilbash, and Sabina Alkire, 157–200. New York: Cambridge University Press, 2008.

Comin, Flavio, Mozaffar Qizilbash, and Sabina Alkire, eds. *The Capability Approach: Concepts, Measures, and Applications.* New York: Cambridge University Press, 2008.

Cooper, John M. "Two Theories of Justice." *Proceedings and Addresses of the American Philosophical Association* 74:2 (November 2000): 3–27.

Crocker, David A., and Ingrid Robeyns. "Capability and Agency." In *Amartya Sen*, edited by Christopher Morris, 60–90. New York: Cambridge University Press, 2010.

Damasio, Antonio. *The Feeling of What Happens: The Body and Emotion in the Making of Consciousness.* New York: Harcourt, 1999.

Daniels, Norman. "Equality of What: Welfare, Resources, or Capabilities?" *Philosophy and Phenomenological Research* 50, supplement (1990): 273–96.

———. *Just Health: Meeting Health Needs Fairly.* New York: Cambridge University Press, 2008.

D'Entreves, A. P. *Natural Law.* New York: Humanities Press, 1964.

Diamond, Jared. *Collapse: How Societies Choose to Fail or Succeed.* New York: Viking, 2005.

Diener, Ed, and Robert Biswas-Diener. *Happiness: Unlocking the Mysteries of Psychological Wealth.* Oxford: Blackwell, 2008.

Doris, John M. *Lack of Character: Personality and Moral Behavior.* New York: Cambridge University Press, 2002.

———, ed., and the Moral Psychology Research Group. *The Moral Psychology Handbook.* New York: Oxford University Press, 2010.

Dworkin, Ronald. *Taking Rights Seriously.* Cambridge, MA: Harvard University Press, 1977.

———. "What Is Equality? Part 1: Equality of Welfare." *Philosophy and Public Affairs* 10 (1981a): 185–245

———. "What Is Equality? Part 2: Equality of Resources." *Philosophy and Public Affairs* 10 (1981b): 283–345.

Elster, Jon. "Norms of Revenge." *Ethics* 100:4 (1990): 862–85.

Emanuel, Ezekiel J. *The Ends of Human Life: Medical Ethics in a Liberal Polity.* Cambridge, MA: Harvard University Press, 1991.

Fleischacker, Samuel. *A Short History of Distributive Justice.* Cambridge, MA: Harvard University Press, 2006.

Frede, Michael. *Essays in Ancient Philosophy.* Minneapolis: University of Minnesota Press, 1987.

Fuller, Lon. "Positivism and Fidelity to Law: A Reply to Professor Hart." *Harvard Law Review* 71:4 (1958): 630–72.

———. *The Morality of Law.* New Haven: Yale University Press, 1964.

Gewirth, Alan. *Reason and Morality.* Chicago: University of Chicago Press, 1978.

———. *Human Rights.* Chicago: University of Chicago Press, 1982.

Gottlieb, Paula. *The Virtue of Aristotle's Ethics.* New York: Cambridge University Press, 2009.

Graham, George. *The Disordered Mind: An Introduction to the Philosophy of Mind and Mental Illness.* New York: Routledge, 2010.

Graver, Margaret. *Stoicism and Emotion.* Chicago: University of Chicago Press, 2007.

Haidt, Jonathan. *The Happiness Hypothesis.* New York: Basic Books, 2006.

Hardin, Russell. *Morality within the Limits of Reason*. Chicago: University of Chicago Press, 1988.

———. *Indeterminacy and Society*. Princeton: Princeton University Press, 2003.

Hart, H. L. A. "Positivism and the Separation of Law and Morals." *Harvard Law Review* 71:4 (1958): 593–629.

———. *The Concept of Law*. Oxford: Clarendon Press, 1961.

———. "Prolegomenon to the Principles of Punishment." In his *Punishment and Responsibility*. New York: Oxford University Press, 1968.

———. "Rawls on Liberty and Its Priority." *University of Chicago Law Review* 40 (1973): 543–55.

Haybron, Daniel M. *The Pursuit of Unhappiness*. New York: Oxford University Press, 2008.

Held, Virginia. *The Ethics of Care: Personal, Political, Global*. New York: Oxford University Press, 2005.

Herman, Barbara. "Agency, Attachment, and Difference." *Ethics* 101:4 (1991): 775–97.

———. *The Practice of Moral Judgment*. Cambridge, MA: Harvard University Press, 1993.

Hierocles. In Ilaria Ramelli, *Hierocles the Stoic: Elements of Ethics, Fragments, and Excerpts*. Translated by David Konstan. Atlanta: Society of Biblical Literature, 2009.

Hobbes, Thomas. *Leviathan*, Chapter XIII.

Hofrichter, Richard. *Health and Social Justice: Politics, Ideology, and Inequity in the Distribution of Disease*. San Francisco: Jossey-Bass, 2003.

Humber, James M., and Robert F. Almeder, eds. *What Is Disease?* Totowa, NJ: Humana Press, 1997.

Hume, David. *Enquiry concerning the Principles of Morals*, pt. 1, sec. 3, "Of Justice."

———. *A Treatise of Human Nature*, bk. 3, pt. 2, sec. 2.

Hurka, Thomas. *Virtue, Vice, and Value*. New York: Oxford University Press, 2001.

———. *The Best Things in Life: A Guide to What Really Matters*. New York: Oxford University Press, 2011.

Jahoda, Marie. *Current Concepts of Positive Mental Health*. Joint Commission on Mental Illness and Health Monograph Series No. 1. New York: Basic Books, 1958.

Kahneman, Daniel. *Judgment under Uncertainty: Heuristics and Biases*. New York: Cambridge University Press, 2001.

———. *Thinking, Fast and Slow*. New York: Farrar, Straus and Giroux, 2011.

Kashdan, T. B. et al. "Reconsidering Happiness: The Costs of Distinguishing between Hedonics and Eudaimonia." *Journal of Positive Psychology* 3 (2008): 219–33.

Kaufman, Charlie, writer. *Being John Malkovich* [film]. 2000.

Kekes, John. *The Human Condition*. New York: Oxford University Press, 2010.

Keyes, Cory L. M. "Toward a Science of Mental Health." In *Oxford Handbook of Positive Psychology*, 2nd ed., edited by C. R. Snyder and Shane J. Lopez, 89–96. New York: Oxford University Press, 2009.

Keyes, Corey L. M., and Joseph G. Grzywacz. "Complete Health: Prevalence and Predictors among US Adults in 1995." *American Journal of Health Promotion* 17:2 (2002): 122–31.

———. "Toward Health Promotion: Physical and Social Behaviors in Complete Health." *American Journal of Health Behavior* 28 (2004): 299–511.

Keyes, Corey L. M., and Julia Annas. "Feeling Good and Functioning Well: Distinctive Concepts in Ancient Philosophy and Contemporary Science." *Journal of Positive Psychology* 4 (2009): 197–201.

Kittay, Eva. *Love's Labor: Essays on Women, Equality, and Dependency* New York: Routledge, 1998.

Korsgaard, Christine M. *The Sources of Normativity*. New York: Cambridge University Press, 1996.

———. *The Constitution of Agency: Essays on Practical Reason and Moral Psychology*. New York: Oxford University Press, 2008.

Landreth, Andrew. "The Emerging Theory of Motivation." In *The Oxford Handbook of Philosophy and Neuroscience*, edited by John Bickle, 381–418. New York: Oxford University Press, 2009.

Lelli, Sarah. "Operationalising Sen's Capability Approach: The Influence of the Selected Technique." In *The Capability Approach: Concepts, Measures, and Applications*, edited by Flavio Comin, Mozaffar Qizilbash, and Sabina Alkire, 310–61. New York: Cambridge University Press, 2008.

Lidz, Theodore. *The Person: His and Her Development throughout the Lifecycle*, rev. ed. New York: Basic Books, 1983.

MacIntyre, Alastair. *After Virtue*, 1st ed.1981; 3rd ed. 2007. South Bend: University of Notre Dame Press, 2007.

Maslow, Abraham. *Motivation and Personality*. New York: Harper, 1954.

Milgram, Stanley. *Obedience to Authority*. New York: HarperCollins, 1974.

Morris, Christopher, ed. *Amartya Sen*. New York: Cambridge University Press, 2010.

Nagel, Thomas. "What Is It like to Be a Bat?" In *Mortal Questions*, 165–80. New York: Cambridge University Press, 1983.

———. *The View from Nowhere*. New York: Oxford University Press, 1986.

Noddings, Nel. *Caring: A Feminine Approach to Ethics and Moral Education*, 1st ed. 1984; updated ed. 2003. Berkeley: University of California Press, 2003.

Nussbaum, Martha C. *The Therapy of Desire*. Princeton: Princeton University Press, 1994.

———. *Women and Human Development: The Capabilities Approach*. New York: Cambridge University Press, 2000.

———. *Upheavals of Thought*. New York: Cambridge University Press, 2001.

———. *Frontiers of Justice*. Cambridge, MA: Belknap Press of Harvard University Press, 2007.

———. *Creating Capabilities: The Human Development Approach*. Cambridge, MA: Belknap Press of Harvard University Press, 2011.

Okin, Susan Moller. *Gender, Justice, and the Family*. New York: Basic Books, 1989.

Patterson, Orlando. *Slavery and Social Death: A Comparative Study*. Cambridge, MA: Harvard University Press, 1992.

Perelman, C. *Justice*. New York: Random House, 1967.

Peterson, Christopher, and Martin Seligman, eds. *Character Strengths and Virtues: A Handbook and Classification*. New York: Oxford University Press, 2004.

Pettit, Philip. "Freedom in the Spirit of Sen." In *The Capability Approach: Concepts, Measures, and Applications*, edited by Christopher Morris, 91–114. New York: Cambridge University Press, 2010.

Phillips, Derek. *Looking Backward: A Critical Appraisal of Communitarian Thought*. Princeton: Princeton University Press, 1993.

Pinker, Steven. *The Better Angels of Our Nature: Why Violence Has Declined*. New York: Viking, 2011.

Powers, Madison, and Ruth Faden. *Social Justice: The Moral Foundations of Public Health and Health Policy*. New York: Oxford University Press, 2006.

Rasmussen, Kasper Lippert. "Justice and Bad Luck." In the *Stanford Encyclopedia of Philosophy* (Online), 2009. Accessed 9/17/ 2011.

Rawls, John. *A Theory of Justice*. Cambridge, MA: Belknap Press of Harvard University Press, 1971.

——. "The Idea of Public Reason Revisited." In *The Law of Peoples; with The Idea of Public Reason Revisited*, 131–80. Cambridge, MA: Harvard University Press, 1999.

Roemer, John. *Equality of Opportunity*. Cambridge, MA: Harvard University Press, 1998.

Royal Anthropological Institute of Great Britain and Ireland. "Political Organization." In *Notes and Queries on Anthropology*, 6th ed., 132–57. London: Routledge and Kegan Paul, 1951. See Chapter V.

Ryan, Richard M., and Veronika Huta. "Wellness as Healthy Functioning or Wellness as Happiness: The Importance of Eudaimonic Thinking." *Journal of Positive Psychology* 4 (2009): 202–4.

Sandel, Michael. *Liberalism and the Limits of Justice*. New York: Cambridge University Press, 1982.

Scanlon, T. M. "Contractualism and Utilitarianism." In *Utilitarianism and Beyond*, edited by Amartya Sen and Bernard Williams, 103–28. New York: Cambridge University Press, 1982.

——. *What We Owe to Each Other*. Cambridge, MA: Harvard University Press, 1998.

Segall, Shlomi. *Health, Luck, and Justice*. Princeton: Princeton University Press, 2010.

Sen, Amartya. "Well-Being, Agency, and Freedom" (Dewey Lectures, 1984). *Journal of Philosophy* 82:4 (1985): 169–221.

——. *The Idea of Justice*. Cambridge, MA: Belknap Press of Harvard University Press, 2009.

Sen, Amartya, and Martha Nussbaum, eds. *Quality of Life*. Oxford: Clarendon Press, 1993.

Silvers, Anita, David Wasserman, and Mary B. Mahowald, with an afterword by Lawrence Becker. *Disability, Difference, Discrimination: Perspectives on Justice in Bioethics and Public Policy*. Totowa, NJ: Rowman and Littlefield, 1998.

Schmidt am Busch, Hans-Christoph, and Christopher F. Zurn, eds. *The Philosophy of Recognition: Historical and Contemporary Perspectives*. Lanham, MD: Lexington Books, 2010.

Snyder, C. R., and Shane J. Lopez, eds. *Oxford Handbook of Positive Psychology*, 2nd ed. New York: Oxford University Press, 2009.

Symposium on Disability. *Ethics* 116:1 (October 2005), with contributions from Lawrence Becker, Anita Silvers and Leslie Francis, Jeff McMahon, Eva Kittay, David Wasserman, and N. Ann Davis.

Thaler, Richard H., and Cass Sunstein. *Nudge: Improving Decisions about Health, Wealth, Happiness.* New Haven: Yale University Press, 2008.

Turnbull, Colin. *The Mountain People.* New York: Simon and Schuster, 1972. Touchstone edition, 1987.

United States v. Holmes 26 F.Cas. 360 (1842).

Vaillant, George. "Mental Health." *American Journal of Psychiatry* 160 (2003): 1373–84.

———. *Spiritual Evolution: A Scientific Defense of Faith.* New York: Broadway Books, 2008.

Vallentyne, Peter. "Brute Luck, Option Luck, and Equality of Initial Opportunities." *Ethics* 112 (2002): 529–57.

———, ed. *Distribution of What?* Vol. 4 of *Equality and Justice.* New York: Routledge, 2003.

———. "Sen on Sufficiency, Priority, and Equality." In *Amartya Sen,* edited by Christopher Morris, 138–69. New York: Cambridge University Press, 2010.

Walzer, Michael. *Spheres of Justice.* New York: Basic Books, 1983.

Wilkinson, Toby. *The Rise and Fall of Ancient Egypt.* New York: Random House, 2011.

Williams, Bernard. "The Idea of Equality." In *Philosophy, Politics and Society,* Second Series, edited by Peter Laslett and W.G. Runciman, 110–31. Oxford: Blackwell, 1962.

Wolff, Jonathan, and Avner de-Shalit. *Disadvantage.* New York: Oxford University Press, 2007.

World Health Organization. *Constitution.* Basic Documents: http://www.who.int/governance/eb/who_constitution_en.pdf. Accessed 06/24/2011.

———. *Mental Health: New Understanding, New Hope.* Geneva, Switzerland: World Health Organization, 2001.

Yates, D. W. "Scoring Systems for Trauma." *British Medical Journal* 301 (1990): 1091–94.

Zygun, David et al. "SOFA Is Superior to MOD Score for the Determination of Non-neurologic Dysfunction in Patients with Severe Traumatic Brain Injury." *Critical Care* 10 (2006): 115.

Index